My New Family

My New Family

Scott A. Milliman Sr.

iUniverse, Inc.
New York Lincoln Shanghai

My New Family

iUniverse books may be ordered through booksellers or by contacting:

iUniverse
2021 Pine Lake Road, Suite 100
Lincoln, NE 68512
www.iuniverse.com
1-800-Authors (1-800-288-4677)

ISBN-13: 978-0-595-36602-6 (pbk)
ISBN-13: 978-0-595-81030-7 (ebk)
ISBN-10: 0-595-36602-3 (pbk)
ISBN-10: 0-595-81030-6 (ebk)

Printed in the United States of America

Contents

Dad,

I know you would be proud of me, I miss you,

You're Son,
Scott.

"What is My New Family?"

It may seem hard to believe for most of the population to believe, but each and every day My New Family grows in number. Sometimes I get a hundred brothers and sisters each day. Sometimes I may only get fifty of each, but in any case Yes, My New Family continues to grow each day.

Growing up as a child, you would expect that growing up you would only be concerned with whether or not Billy could play baseball with you after school or if Susan liked you because she looked and smiled at you today. Remember these feelings? There was always homework to do and phone calls to make. Come on and face it, you were a kid, and what does a kid want? Yes, he wants to play and enjoy life. Do you actually know what life is when you are a child? Do you think about real life as just time to play and go to school? Yes, most children do, but to some children there is a time where they sit back and try to remember all their brothers' and sisters' names because it's hard. The list of their names gets longer and longer with each day. It is these children who face what life is truly about: and that's for them waking up each and everyday fighting a disease that has come over them, that being cancer.

Some children don't know what it feels like to play with Billy or smile at Susan; their lives are consumed by trying to stay alive.

You may never know and probably wont know all your brothers' and sisters' names within this family. The name of this family is *cancer victims*. This family name is stronger than any family you will ever meet; the Gottis, Kennedy's, Brushes, and Smiths don't even compete with your family's strength and abilities. You will play a different game than Billy; you will play the game of life...and the expectant look from Susan might actually be a look from your doctor. It's that look that you won't forget, and it's that look that you feel like you're in love with.

It was July 16, 2002, when I met my first sister of My New Family. I had just returned home from having an MRI of my brain at a local hospital. Over the past thirteen months or so, I had been having what I called "attacks." As my vision would become blurry, and I would get tunnel vision. After each of these incidents, I would get a very bad acid taste in my mouth. My doctor kept insisting that I was having a panic or anxiety attack because I was a police officer. I must stop talking about this doctor now, because of possible litigation against him. A second doctor referred me to a neurologist. I scheduled a visit, and after examining me within seconds the neurologist wanted me to go for an brain MRI. I was still feeling pretty good about myself then came that awful news after the mri, that I had a large tumor on the right side of my brain.

I looked at the radiologist and said, "Yeah right, you got the wrong name on the MRI sheets."

It turned out to be the right name, and I was floored. I didn't have a clue on about what to do. My wife and I came home, and we met our neighbors, who have always been great to have. I got a hug from Linda, who hugged me after she heard about the results, and I immediately felt a connection. It was a weird, internal type feeling that made me somewhat more comfortable.

As she pulled away from me, she looked at me and said, "Scott, you can handle it. I went through breast cancer recently."

I looked at Linda and felt so badly for her. I knew she had been sick for a while, but I didn't really know why. Here my new sister was hurting, I didn't even help her when she was hurt, and now she is helping me? Linda, I wish I knew more at that time. I would have been honored to help you; you live just two doors down from me. You made me feel more confident this first afternoon after discovery that I had cancer.

I had surgery six days later on July 22 at Rush St. Luke's Medical Center in Chicago, Illinois. I can't say enough for Dr. Byrnes and the entire staff. They were top-of-the-line in my book. The surgery was supposed to last four hours, but instead it lasted nine and a half. I was awake through the whole surgery, and during this time I met another sister, Jessica, who in reality was my daughter Jessica, but I kept seeing her in close contact with my face yelling, "Don't give up. Don't let me down." I had these thoughts the entire time through surgery, even thou actually the the person looking into my eyes this whole time during surgery was a Doctor wearing goggles, looking into my eyes every second, and every minute or so he would have me move left shoulder, then arm, and leg, making sure I still have movement. I couldn't see the doctors eyes through the goggles, but sure heard every word my daughter had spoken to me before about not giving up. This was very clear.

It was the next morning, while I was in the Intensive Care Unit, that I heard about another family member. I was visited early in the morning by a doctor. He checked me out and said I was doing very good. He then said that he had to go perform now, for another surgery. I then opened my eyes fully, looked at him, and asked him what type of surgery it was. Something was telling me to ask more questions. He said that a small child had come in, and that the child's tumor had already affected his motor skills, and that it was very difficult to operate on. He then left the room to go to surgery. I immediately put my hands together as tight as I could with the intravenous tubes and everything else attached to them and asked the Lord to save my brother or sister. It bothered me all day. The next morning the doctor came back into my room, and before he could even check me out, all I wanted to know was how my brother was doing. He looked at me kind of strangely and appeared confused. I asked him how the child was doing from yesterday's surgery was doing, and I saw the doctor's eyes fill up with tears some what. He changed the subject by checking me out. I knew then that I had lost a very important family member. I looked at my wife, who had been sleeping next to me since surgery, and she knew that the news wasn't good either. I decided to write this book—not for me—but for all my brothers and sisters out there. I wish that I could know each and every one. Yes, you have the Larsons, Freidmans, and the Smiths, but those are only last names…we are all one family, the cancer victims of the world.

My New Family members are from all walks of life. I don't care about what color you are, your origin, your religion, or where you live...you all are a part of my family. To me it doesn't matter if you have a million dollars, or if you are living on a cardboard box under a train station. My New Family will remain intact, and no person or power will be able to separate us. To my brother who is homeless, you should be able to play ball just as much with Billy, as you my brother who lives in a mansion, and lots or rooms. I could have sisters and brothers who range in age from one year old up to a hundred or more years old. We all are in this family together.

We must, and will be able to help each one of us other; it could be by sending an e-mail, a get-well card, a box of cookies, candy, pie, or just simply taking each other out for a ride to look at some sights. For those of us who are in financial need, we must figure out ways to help each other. This will be our new family motto. We suffer enough, but we can help the suffering by helping others. We lost so many family members in the past who we took life for granted—like Phillip Montalbano and Walter Payton. I could only wish that I was a part of this family before, or had the love to help. It's sad that I had to view such a tragedy as this to get My New Family to bloom. I lost my father, John, to diabetes complications when I was young, and then I lost my brother, John Jr., to the same disease.

I had no ancestors affected by cancer. I'm not sure why God picked me, but I think it has to do with my state of mind, my willingness to always help others. I don't sit back and say, "Oh, why me?" or "It's not fair." I look at this as an opportunity in my life that can open the doors for others to see that there is life out there for all of us; we just have to try a bit harder to be able to help others. To my sisters with breast cancer, keep pushing and don't give up, and for those sisters not yet affected, please take the self-tests to help in the early detection of this terrible cancer.

In the beginning, I tried to figure out how many years back My New Family tree goes, or where it began to grow. From what I have seen and heard, our brothers and sisters have been suffering for a long time…in my eyes—way too long. Many years. Like hundreds of years to long. I begin this book by looking at cancer research and how the ability to detect cancer has progressed. Basically, I came to my own conclusion that we have not gone to many forward years enough, into stopping this. Out of despite all these years of research, not to mention how much money has been spent. For or set aside for research to stop this deadly spread. I sometimes think of all my brothers' and sisters' names, and then I drive by a cemetery and look at their names. I think about the lives they had been living here with us. It makes me really concerned about the progress of cancer research. Why are so many of us are falling by the wayside so quickly? Are we, as victims, doing everything we can to help this program? By the time you reach the name of *victim*, it's too late in my book to say you are helping the program or helping with research.

I say these comments not because I am looking at the fact that I just have cancer. I'm not saying, this because of "Why me?" I'm saying, "Why My New Family members? Why?"

There are more than 8,000 scientists working on a cure for cancer today. More than 8,000. Are any of these scientists my brothers or sisters? They should be. They would have a stronger drive to find a cure. I am not against all the scientists and research centers. .no im not. I do support that they have helped in ways to build our immune system, and for some area or forms of cancer they have allowed us to live longer. Live longer? Do they know how some of my family members live longer? What it takes for them to complete each day? Yes, each day that we continue to breathe is a blessing. But for a lot of us, it's a large amount of pain and suffering. But we exchange the pain and suffering for waking up one more day.

Some of these scientists have won Nobel Prizes and other awards. They have been saluted by the Academy of Scientists and other organizations. Well, that's all fine and nice, but usually when a person gets rewarded for something, it's because they have finished something or have done something so remarkable. I'm not taking away from any of these awards from the scientists, but I would just like to know one thing….one thing….did you find a cure for cancer?

I know you (the scientists have helped in looking for a cure for My New Family in alternative medicines, and even some pre-cancer prevention therapies. But have these proved as valuable as finding the actual cure for cancer?

For instance, my mother, Lorraine Montalbano, who has been a true blessing to me and will continue to be for My New Family, suggested to me how to organize cancer research across the country. One scientist in Florida is working on the same thing as a scientist in California. Mom says baloney. Put these scientists together and let them work together. For example, all scientists working on breast cancer should work together at the same university. And guess what, by working together, they can find the cure for it, and help each other. Brain cancer research might be centered in West Virginia (a very special state for me, as I will explain later). Too much money is being spread around the world in research, and a lot of people are earning fat pay checks trying to find a cure. Well, if you are trying so hard, let's see the game plan....Oh no, that's right, you are on the offensive side—not the defensive side like My New Family is. My family would ask each victim questions about the past and try to find similarities. I was not asked a single question about my history. Questions should be asked: "Have you had any X-rays? If so, how many? Any dental work completed? If so, what, and what was used, what type of material? Do you smoke marijuana? If so, how much? Do you grow your own vegetable garden?" Start a process of elimination!

I was so excited to hear that after my surgery, a scientific team was going to examine my tumor. I was so happy. This could hopefully help My New Family. I called back a week later and was told that my tumor, who I named "Hank," was currently set at 180 degrees below zero. I am not a scientist, but close (a police officer, OK, maybe not close then), but I did ask the scientist what he would be testing for.? He advised me that he would be examining the DNA. I said, "Wow, that sounds like some cool stuff," and asked him about making the tumor they took out to try and make it grow again. They could find out what feeds these thing and causes it to grow. He said yes, he would try.

I then waited four weeks and decided to call the scientist back to see how Hank was doing. He told me that he hadn't started anything yet, which I understood because he was probably busy with other tumors. Before hanging up, I asked him to test Hank for certain proteins and also microwave rays to see if the tumor reacts or grows. To my surprise,heart aching response the scientist told me that he was unable to do this because Hank was frozen.

The scientist told me, "If you wanted this procedure done, you should have told me earlier so we could have preserved the tumor differently."

"Now wait a minute," I said. "It's not like we don't have enough going on before surgery to worry about this too. No one ever mentioned this to me before."

So this is where My New Family should become active, paid employees in cancer research. If the scientist himself was a victim or the family member of one, I'm sure he would have thought of this process, but without that family internal love and bond, he let another one go by.

"Maybe we will test others in the future this way," he said.

I hung up feeling so much hurt, knowing that my Hank could have made a lot of My New Family happy because we could have tested it for growth and tested various methods to kill Hank.

From what I have seen and experienced myself, most of my brothers and sisters have financial troubles. With all the doctor's visits, medicine, car trips, and food, I think my family needs to be gainfully employed at these research centers. To help others as well. They have the drive and the will to get the job done. Why? Because they are family!

Besides the medical problems that we go through as a family, like I said before the financial problems that we have to face are sometimes just as hard as our fight to cure cancer. I know I said it before, but I must stress my strong belief that those in the family could find jobs within the research groups if all the research groups become more organized, and generally located by type or form of cancer. I don't care if it's ten or one hundred of my brothers and sisters who secure a paying job at the centers; it's better than not being able to work at all, and we all would benefit more from this because all these family members have a strong cause and will to think, and work harder for finding—or assisting in finding—a cause and cure for cancer, more than someone who is just collecting a hefty paycheck every two weeks. My family would feel a lot better to-do anything to be gainfully employed and helping in this cause. A lot of cancer victims end up losing their jobs because of cancer, time off, and doctor's visits. Heck, I have been told about so many people who don't return to work, their same jobs, because of their battle with cancer. I wonder if employers ever think that they might be able to look down on someone and treat them more roughly just because they have cancer? I sure hope not we can still work, even if it's not at one hundred percent. We can still do it, Mr. or Mrs. Employer!

Fear and Hope.

Well, let me tell you something, Mr. Employer. There are two big emotions that My New Family must think about: fear and hope. We will always have fear. Unless you have had your breast removed, your colon taken out, your liver replaced, or had lung surgery, brain surgery, testicular, ovarian, or any of the other forms of cancer-related problems, you will never know what the word *fear* means. This type of fear is the worst feeling that a person could go through..during this type of fear, I It tends take control of your body, and you have to fight hard against it. You must.

During the fear mode of our lives, we each go through and a different form of fear, everyone deals with it differently. Family and friends can be the best medicine for fear. They'll be there for you when you need them and even at times when you think you don't. My fear hit me very hard. I was a big, tough, well-built police officer for the sheriff's office. Up until I found out about my tumor, I thought fear was pulling up on a call and seeing citizens running away from a house or apartment where somebody is firing a gun and running past the citizens as they are fleeing. All the while, your mind is telling you, "Wait a minute, if they are running away, why am I running in?" and not away then? I

It wasn't until my brother, Kurt, who I love and admire so much, came to my home the morning after I found out about the tumor. It was here that I felt a different type of fear, but yet so similar in words. Kurt and my nephew Bobby grabbed me, and Kurt looked at me and said, "Come on, Scott, we will go into this together."

I no longer felt that I was running into that home by myself, but rather that I was running into that home with an armored tank. It made me realize that, yes, we can deal with fear and go on. The night before this, I had kept reminding myself that I had a lovely wife, Wendy, of nineteen years, a beautiful daughter, Jessica, two great, and I mean great, sons, Jon and Scott Jr. This same night I took my service weapon apart into as many pieces as I could, hoping that I might forgot how to put it back together.

"It is just a fear that I had to deal with," I kept telling myself. "The tumor is there. It's reality; now just let's deal with it. It is what it is. Let's go and fight it."

The second word that I talked about was *hope*. What is hope? I found the definition of hope by waking up into ICU and counting how many cylinder bricks were there that made up the wall that I was now looking at from the bed, I knew that at this point I had made it out of surgery. Even though I was awake for the nine hours of the surgery, *hope* was this new word that I had. But it wasn't a big word or emotion to me. A couple of weeks later, I went to Evanston-Northwestern Hospital in Evanston to see Dr. Paleologos. I walked into the waiting room with Wendy, Kurt, Karyn, and my mother, Lorraine. I looked in the waiting room, and there were at least eighteen brothers and sisters sitting there waiting for various cancer treatments, some in wheelchairs, some using walkers, some looking very tired and sick. But one thing out from the beginning, they all looked at me and smiled. I didn't know any of these cancer victims, neither did they know each other. But those smiles, as I smiled back at them, made us a part of the family. We all knew and felt the unity that we would share. It didn't matter that some were fifteen years old and others were in their eighties. We didn't care or even think like that; we were that new family.

Now looking back at the word *hope*, I see I took it for granted early on with my struggle. I have such a demanding and caring sister named Karyn. As soon as I broke the news, or I should say Wendy had to talk to my mom because I couldn't get the words out of my mouth when I found out about the tumor, Karyn began to work hard to find me a hospital, and a diagnosis. Karyn has her own home healthcare treatment business, so she has seen a lot of the similar situations after surgery, as I would soon to find out. But I knew with Karyn working away at it that I didn't have to worry. About the end of it. I trusted in my sister, and she proved me right time after time. She replaced the word *fear* with the word *hope*. I made up my mind that right or wrong, that I would always go with her advice, and I knew that I would never look down on it negatively if anything did happen during surgery. She gave me hope, and where would I have been without hope?

The small county hospital by my house had maybe done one brain surgery in five years. No, she knew what had to be done and how to do it.

Yes, My New Family, I want you to meet your new mother, Lorraine, your new sister, Karyn, Wendy, and your new brother, Kurt. They don't have the disease we have, but they are still your family. They will rejoice and be so thrilled to have you in their family.

Hope doesn't have to be just for those with cancer. No, it's not limited to the family. Hope can be shared by all and can help those with cancer or any other illness. All you have to do is join My New Family and help wherever you can. It might be that second policeman running into that house, or trying out your cooking skills, sitting down to find a solution to the financial problems, helping with locating a job or a place to work, or simply taking your brother or sister out for a ride and to show them something maybe they have never seen before—maybe a buffalo, a park, a new street, a pizzeria, anything....Help build that hope. The following few pages, are the actual printed pages that I used in the beginning of writing my book. Some of the pages you might have read already, or about to read. I have included this in my book, because hopefully you will be able to look at the way that I had to type, not nowing before on how to. I typed from my heart and soul. Am I a good speller? Do I use proper grammer? Are the sentences lined up? The hell if I knew, but what I know for sure is that I sat here and typed for all of us, My New Family. Although the editors might have changed a word around, or corrected some of the text, you should be able to see that it's still me typing away.

IT MAY SEEM HARD TO BELIEVE TO MOST OF THE POPULATION,BUT EACH AND EVERY DAY MY FAMILY GROWS IN NUMBERS,SOMETIMES I GET 100 BROTHERS AND OR 100 SISTERS EACH DAY,SOMETIME I MAY GET 50 AND 50 OF EACH,BUT IN ANY CASE YES,MY FAMILY CONTINUES TO GROW EACH DAY.

GROWING UP AS A CHILD,ONE WOULD EXPECT TO BE CONCERN WHETHER OR NOT BILLY CAN PLAY BASEBALL AFTER SCHOOL,OR IF SUSAN LIKES YOU BECAUSE SHE LOOKED AND SMILED AT YOU TODAY..THERES ALWAYS HOMEWORK TO DO,AND PHONCE CALLS TO MAKE..COME ON AND FACE IT,YOUR A KID AND WHAT DOES A KID WANT?..YES,HE WANTS TO PLAY AND ENJOY LIFE..DO YOU ACTUALY KNOW WHAT LIFE IS WHEN YOUR A CHILD?.DO YOU THINK ABOUT REAL LIFE AS JUST TIME TO PLAY AND SCHOOL?..YES,MOST OF CHILDREN DO,BUT TO SOME CHILDREN,THERE IS A TIME WHERE THEY SIT BACK AND TRY TO REMEMBER ALL THIER BROTHERS AND SISTERS NAMES,BECUASE ITS HARD,THE LIST OF THIER NAMES GET LONGER AND LONGER WITH EACH DAY...IT IS THESE CHILDREN THAT FACE WHAT LIFE IS TRULY ABOUT,AND THATS FOR THEM WAKING UP EACH AND EVERYDAY FIGHTING A DISEASE THAT HAS COME OVER THEM,THAT BEING CANCER..TO SOME,THE CHILDREN DONT KNOW WHAT IT FEELS LIKE TO PLAY WITH BILLY,OR SMILE AT SUSAN,THIER LIFE IS CONSUMED BY TRYING TO HAVE LIFE.

YOU MAY NEVER KNOW,AND PROBABLY WONT KNOW ALL YOUR BROTHERS AND SISTERS NAMES WITHIN THIS FAMILY.THE NAME OF THE FAMILY IS CANCER VICTIMS.THE FAMILY NAME IS STRONGER THANY ANY FAMILY YOU WILL EVER MEET,THE GOTTS,KENNEDY'S,BUSHS DONT EVEN COMPETE WITH YOUR FAMILYS STRENGTH AND ABILTIES..YOU WILL PLAY A DIFFERANT GAME THEN BILLY,THE GAME OF LIFE...AND THE LOOK FROM SUSAN MIGHT BE FROM YOUR DOCTOR,ITS THAT LOOK THAT YOU WILL FEEL LIKE YOUR IN LOVE WITH.

IT WAS JULY 16TH,2002 WHEN I MET MY FIRST SISTER OF MY NEW FAMILY..I HAD JUST RETURNED HOME FROM A LOCAL HOSPITAL HAVING A M.R.I OF MY BRAIN..OVER THE PAST 13 MONTH I WAS HAVING WHAT I CALLED "ATTACK",AS MY VISION WOULD BE BLURRY AND TUNNEL VISION AND I WOULD GET A VERY BAD ACID TASTE IN MY MOUTH AFTER EACH OF THESE INCIDENTS.MY DOCTOR KEPT INSISTING THAT I WAS HAVING A PANIC ATTACK OR ANIXITY ATTACK BECAUSE I WAS A POLICE OFFICER.I WOULD PASS EVERY TEST,AND WAS VERY AHRD ON KEEPING ME HEALTHY BY RUNNING AND WEIGHT LIFTING,AND I DIDNT FEEL LIKE I WAS HAVING ANY PANIC ATTACKS.I FINALY WAS SENT TO A NUEROLIGIST BY ANOTHER DOCTOR WHO SCHEDULED THE MRI.I WORKED HARD FOR THE LAST SEVERAL YEARS TO SAVE UP ENOUGH MONEY TO TAKE MY WIFE AND CHILDREN TO DISNEY WORLD.WE CAME BACK ON A THURSDAY,AND WENT TO THE MRI ON THE FOLLOWING TUESDAY.I WAS STILL FEELING VERY GOOD ABOUT MY SELF.THEN CAME THAT AWFUL NEWS AFTER THE MRI WAS TAKEN THAT I HAVE A LARGE BRAIN TUMOR ON THE RIGHT SIDE OF MY BRAIN.I LOOKED AT THE RADIOLISGST AND SAID,"YEH RIGHT,YOU GOT THE WRONG NAME ON THE MRI SHEETS".IT TURNED OUT TO BE THE CORRECT NAME,AND I WAS "FLOORED".DIDNT HAVE A CLUE ON WHAT TO DO.ME AND MY WIFE CAME HOME,AND WE MET OUR NEIGHBORS WHO HAVE ALWAYS BEEN GREAT TO HAVE...I GOT A HUG FROM LAURA CHRISTOPHER AFTER SHE HEARD ABOUT THE RESULTS,AND I IMMEDIATLY FELT A CONNECTION.IT WAS A WIERD INTERNAL TYPE FEELING THAT MADE ME SOMEWHAT MORE COMFORTABLE..AS SHE PULLED AWAY FROM ME,SHE LOOKED AT ME AND SAID"SCOTT,YOU CAN HANDLE IT,I WENT THROUGH A DOUBLE BREAST CANCER TREATMENT RECENTLY..I LOOKED AT LAURA,AND FELT SO BAD FOR HER,AS I KNEW THAT SHE WAS SICK FOR AWILE,BUT DIDNT REALLY KNOW WHY.HERE MY NEW SISTER WAS HURTING,AND I DIDNT EVEN HELP HER WHEN SHE WAS HURT,AND NOW SHE IS HELPING ME?

I HAD SURGERY 6 DAYS LATER ON JULY 22,2002 AT RUSH/ST LUKES MEDICAL IN CHICAGO.I CANT SAY ENOUGH FOR THE SURGEON DR BYRNES,AND THE ENTIRE STAFF.TOP OF THE LINE IN MY BOOKS.THE SURGERY WAS TO BE 4 HRS,BUT WENT 9 AND 1/2 HOURS.I WAS AWAKE DURING THIS WHOLE SURGERY,AND DURING THIS IS WHERE I MET MY SISTER SUSAN,WHO IN REALTY WAS MY DAUGHTER JESSICA,BUT I KEPT SEEING HER IN CLOSE CONTACT WITH MY FACE YELLING"DONT GIVE UP,DONT LET ME DOWN"....

p

IT WAS THE NEXT MORNING, JULY 23RD WHILE I WAS IN THE I.C.U. THAT I MET MY NEXT FAMILY MEMBER..I WAS VISTITED EARLY IN THE MORNING BY DR BYRNES.HE CHECKED ME OUT AND SAID I WAS DOING VERY GOOD.HE THEN SAID THAT HE HAS TO GO NOW FOR ANOTHER SURGERY..I THEN OPENED MY EYES FULLY,LOOKED AT HIM AND ASKED HIM WHAT TYPE OF SURGERY?..SOMETHING WAS TELLING ME TO ASK MORE QUESTIONS.HE SAID THAT A SMALL CHILD HAD CAME IN ,AND THAT THE CHILDS TUMOR HAD ALREADY SPREAD TO HIS MOTOR SKILLS AND WAS VERY DIFFICULT.HE THEN LEFT THE ROOM TO GO TO SURGERY.I IMMEDIATLY PUT MY AHNDS TOGETHER AND ASKED THAT THE LORD SAVE MY BROTHER/OR SISTER..IT BOTHERED ME ALL DAY.THE NEXT MORNING DR BYRNES CAME BACK INTO MY ROOM NOW,AND BEFORE HE COULD EVEN CHECK ME OUT,ALL I WANTED TO KNOW IS HOW MY BROTHER OR SISTER WAS DOING?..HE LOOKED AT ME KINDA OF STANGE,AND APPEARED CONFUSED.I ASKED HIM HOW THE CHILD WAS DOING FROM YESTERDAYS SURGERY,AND ALL I SAW WAS THE DOCTORS EYES FILL UP WITH WATER SOME WHAT,AND HE CHANGE THE STORY BY CHECKING ME OUT.I KNEW THEN THAT I HAD JUST LOST A VERY IMPORTANT FAMILY MEMBER..I LOOKED AT MY WIFE WHO HAD BEEN SLEEPING NEXT TO ME SINCE SURGERY,AND SHE KNEW THAT THE NEWS WASNT GOOD EITHER..I DECIDED TO WRITE THIS BOOK NOT FOR ME,BUT FOR ALL MY BROTHERS AND SISTERS OUT THERE,AND WISH THAT I COULD KNOW EACH AND EVERY ONE,..YES YOU HAVE THE LARSONS,THE FRIEDMANS,THE GLINES,..BUT ITS ONLY A LAST NAME..WE ARE ALL THE FAMILY,THE CANCER VICTIMS OF THE WORLD.

MY NEW FAMILY ARE FROM ALL WALKS OF LIFE..I DONT CARE ABOUT WHAT COLOR YOU ARE,YOUR ORGIN,YOUR RELIGION,OR WHERE YOU LIVE,..YOU ALL ARE A PART OF MY FAMILY.....................TO ME IT DOESNT MATTER IF YOU HAVE A MILLION DOLLARS,OR IF YOU ARE LIVING ON A CARDBOARD BOX UNDER A TRAIN STATION,MY NEW FAMILY WILL REMIAN INTACT,NO ONE OR POWER WILL BE ABLE TO SEPERATE US APART..TO MY BROTHER WHO IS HOMELESS,YOU SHOULD BE ABLE TO PLAY BALL JUST AS MUCH WITH BILLY AS YOU MY BROTHER WHO LIVE IN A MANSION,AND LOTS OF ROOMS..I COULD HAVE A SISTER OR BROTHER THAT IS 1 YEAR OLD,OR UP TO 100 OR MORE YEARS OLD.WE ALL ARE IN THIS FAMILY TOGETHER.

WE MUST,AND WILL BE ABLE TO HELP EACH ONE OF US.IT COULD BE FROM A EMAIL,A GET WELL CARD,BOX OF COOKIES OR CANDY,PIE,YOU JUST SIMPLY TAKING EACH OTHER OUT FOR A RIDE AND LOOK AT SOME SITES.FOR THOSE OF US THAT ARE FIANCIAL IN NEED,WE MUST FIGURE OUT WAYS TO HELP EACH OTHER.THIS WILL BE OUR NEW FAMILY MOTTO.WE SUFFER ENOUGH,BUT WE CAN HELP THE SUFFERING BY HELPING OTHERS...WE LOST SEVERAL FAMILY MEMBERS IN THE PAST THAT WE TOOK LIFE FOR GRANTED,LIKE PHILLIP MONTALBANO AND WALTER PAYTON.I COULD ONLY WISH THAT I WAS A PART OF THIS FAMILY BEFORE,OR HAD THE LOVE TO HELP..ITS SAD THAT I HAD TO VIEW SUCH TRADEGY AS THIS TO GET MY NEW FAMILY TO BLOOM...I LOST MY FATHER JOHN WHEN I WAS YOUNG TO DIABETIS COMPLICATIONS,AND THEN I LOST MY BROTHER JOHN JR TO THE SAME DESIASE.

I HAVE NO PASTGENERATIONS THAT CANCER HAS EFFECTED THEM.IM NOT SURE WHY THE GOD PICKED ME,BUT I THINK IT HAS TO DO WITH MY STATE OF MIND,THE WILLINGNESS TO ALWAYS HELP OTHERS.I DONT SIT BACK AND SAY"OH,WHY ME""OR "ITS NOT FAIR".I LOOK AT THIS AS THE OPENING OF MY LIFE THAT CAN OPEN THE DOORS TO OTHERS TO SE THAT THERE IS LIFE OUT THERE FOR ALL OF US,WE JUST HAVE TO PUSH AND TRY A BIT HARDER,AND TO BE ABLE TO HELP OTHERS..TO MY NEW SISTERS WHO BREAST CANCER HAS REALLY TAKEN A COURSE ON,KEEPING PUSHING,DONT GIVE UP,AND FOR THE OTHER SISTERS,PLEASE TAKE THE SELF TESTS TO HELP IN EARLY DETECTION OF THIS TERRIBLE CANCER.

IN THE BEGINNING.

I HAVE TRIED TO FIGURE OUT HOW LONG IN YEARS DOES MY NEW FAMILY TREE GO,OR WHERE IT BEGAN TO GROW?...FROM WHAT I HAVE SEEN AND HEARD,OUR BROTHERS AND SISTERS HAVE BEEN SUFFERING FOR ALONG TIME..IN MY EYES,WAY TO MANY YEARS,LIKE HUNDREDS OF YEARS TO LONG..I BEGIN THIS BY LOOKING AT THE RESEARCH OF CANCER,AND HOW IT HAS PROGRESSED TO A LEVEL OF DETECTION IN CURRENT DAYS..BASICALLY I CAME TO MY OWN CONCLUSION THAT WE HAVE NOT GONE TO MANY FORWARD YEARS INTO STOPPING THIS..OUT OF ALL THESE YEARS OF RESEARCH,AND NOT EVEN NAMING HOW MUCH MONEY HAS BEEN SPENT FOR OR SET ASIDE FOR RESEARCH TO STOP THIS DEADLY SPREAD,I SOMETIMES THINK OF ALL MY BROTHRES AND SISTERS NAMES,AND THEN DRUVE BY A CEMATARY AND LOOK AT THIER NAMES AND THE YOUNG LIVES THAT THEY HAD LIVING HERE WITH US,MAKES ME REAL CONCERNED ABOUT THIS RESEARCH..WHY SO MANY OF US ARE FALLING TO THE WAY SIDE SO QUICK?..ARE WE AS VICTIMS DOING EVERYTHING WE CAN TO HELP THIS PROGRAM?..WELL,BY THE TIME YOU REACH THE NAME OF "VICTIM",ITS TO LATE IN MY BOOKS TO SAY YOU ARE HELPING THE PROGRAM!..OR HELPING WITH RESEARCH!...

I SAY THESE COMMENTS NOT BECAUSE I AM LOOKING AT THE FACT THAT I HAVE CANCER,NO...IM NOT SAYING "OH WHY ME"...NO,IM SAYING WHY MY NEW FAMILY,WHY?

THERE ARE WELL OVER 3,000 SCIENTISTS WORKING ON A CURE FOR CANCER TODAY.WELL OVER 3,000..ARE ANY OF THESE SCIENTISTS MY BROTHERS OR SISTERS?..THEY SHOULD BE.THEN THEY WILL HAVE A STRONGER DRIVE TO FIND THE CURE...I AM NOT AGAINST ALL THE SCIENTISTS AND RESEARCH CENTERS,NO IM NOT...I DO SUPPORT THAT THEY HAVE HELPED IN WAYS TO BUILD OUR IMMUNE SYSTEM,AND IN SOME AREA OR FORMS OF CANCER,THEY HAVE ALLOWED US TO LIVE LONGER..LIVE LONGER?..DO THEY KNOW HOW SOME OF MY FAMILY LIVE LONGER?.WHAT IT TAKES FOR THEM TO COMPLETE EACH DAY?..YES,EACH DAY THAT WE CONTINUE TO BREATH IS A BLESSING,BUT FOR ALOT OF US,ITS A LARGE AMOUNT OF PAIN AND SUFFERING..BUT WE EXCHANGE THE PAIN AND SUFFERING FOR WAKING UP ONE MORE DAY.

SOME OF THESE SCIENTISTS HAVE WON NOBEL AND OTHER AWARDS,HAVE BEEN SALUTED BY ACADEMY OF SCIENTISTS,AND OTHER ORGINIZATIONS....WELL,THATS ALL FINE AND NICE..BUT USUALLY WHEN A PERSON WOULD GET REWARDED FOR SOMETHING,ITS BECAUSE THEY HAVE COMPLETED SOMETHING OR HAS DID SOMETHING SO REMARKABLE..IM NOT TAKING AWAY ANY OF THESE AWARDS FROM THE SCIENTISTS,BUT WOULD JUST LIKE TO KNOW ONE THING,....DID YOU FIND A CURE FOR CANCER?

I KNOW,YOU (THE SCIENTISTS)HAVE HELPED IN AFTER CURE FOR MY NEW FAMILY IN ALTERNTIVE MEDICENS,AND EVEN SOME PRE CANCER PREVENTION THERYS..BUT HAVE THESE PROVED AS VALUABLE SA FINDING THE ACTUAL CURE FOR CANCER..

FOR INSTANCE....BY USING MY MOTHERS LORRAINE MONTALBANO SUGGESTION,WHO AHS BEEN A TRULY BLESSING TO ME,AND WILL CONTINUE TO BE FOR MY NEW FAMILY..MOM SUGGESTED TO ME THAT WITH CANCER RESEARCH,ITS WAY TO SPREAD OUT OVER THE COUNTRY..I SCIENTISTS IN FLORIDA IS WORKING ON THE SAME THING AS A SCIENSTIST IS WORKING ON IN CALIFORNIA....MOM SAYS "BOLANGA"..PUT THESE SCIENTISTS TOGETHER,AND LET THEM WORK TOGETHER..FOR EXAMPLE..FOR BREAST CANCER,ALL SCIENTISTS WILL WORK TOGETHER AT THE A CERTAIN UNIVERISTY,AND GUESS WHAT?..THAT WHAT YOU WILL DO,FIND THE CURE FOR IT AND HELP EACH OTHER..BRAIN CANCER MIGHT BE IN WEST VIRGINIA(A VERY SPECIAL STATE FOR ME,EXPLAIN LATER)...TO MUCH MONEY IS BEING SPREAD AROUND THE WORLD IN RESEARCH,AND ALOT OF PEOPLE MAKING WEALTHY PAYCHECKS BY "TRYING" TO FIND A CURE....WELL,IF YOU WERE TRYING SO HARD ON A CERTAIN AREA,LETS SEE THE GAME PLAN....OH NO,THATS RIGHT,YOUR ON OFFENSE SIDE,NOT DEFENSE LIKE MY FAMILY IS..MY FAMILY WOULD ASK EACH VICTIM QUESTIONS ABOUT THE PAST AND TRY TO FIND A SIMIALIAR INSTANCE..I WAS NOT ASKED A SINGLE QUESTION ABOUT MINE...THERE SHOULD BE QUESTIONS LIKE..HAVE ANY XRAYS?,IF SO HOW MANY..ANY DENTAL WORK,IF SO WHAT,AND WHAT WAS USED?..SMOKE MARIJUANA?.IF SO,HOW MUCH..GROW YOUR OWN GARDEN?..START A PROCESS OF ELIMANTION.

I WAS SO EXCITED TO HEAR THAT AFTER SURGERY,THEY WILL TAKE THE TUMOR AND EXAMINE IT BY A SCIENTIST TEAM..OH BOY,YEA..I WAS SO HAPPY,THEY CAN HOPEFULLY HELP MY NEW FAMILY..I CALLED BACK 1 WEEK LATER,AND WAS TOLD THAT MY TUMOR WHO I NAMED "HANK"WAS CURRENTLY SET AT 180 DEGREES BELOW ZERO...I AM NOT A SCIENTISTS,BUT CLOSE(A POLICE OFFICER)..OK,MAYBE NOT CLOSE THEN........I ASKED THE SCIENTIST WHAT HE WILL BE TESTING FOR??..HE ADVISED ME THAT HE WILL BE TESTING FOR GENE MAKE UP,AND DNA..I SAID WOW,THAT SOUNDS LIKE SOME COOL STUFF,AND ASKED HIM ABOUT MAKING THE TUMOR GROW AGAIN?.HE SAID YES,HE WILL TRY......I THEN WAITED 4 WEEKS,AND DECIDED TO CALL THE SCIENTIST BACK,SEE HOW"HANK"IS DOING..HE TOLD ME THAT HE HASNT STARTED ANYTHING YET,WHICH I UNDERSTAND,HES PROPABLY BUSY WITH OTHER TUMORS..BEFORE HANGING UP WITH HIM,I ASKED HIM THAT WHEN HE BRINGS "HANK"BACK TO GROWTH,TEST HANK FOR CERTAIN PROTEINS AND ALSO MICROWAVES TO SEE IF IT REACTS OR GROWS..TO MY HEART ACKING RESPONSE,THE SCIENTIST TOLD ME THAT HE IS UNABLE TO FEED IT ANY OF THESE REQUESTS,AS BECAUSE OF THE TUMORS CERTAIN FREEZING CONDITION...THE SCIENTIST TOLD ME THEN"IF YOU WANTED THIS PROCESS DONE TO SEE IF IT WOULD GROW WITH CERTAIN THINGS,THATS A DIFFERANT PROCEDURE TO PROTECT THE TUMOR AND YOU WOULD HAVE TOLD ME BEFORE THE SURGERY WAS DONE SO WE CAN PRESERVE THE TUMOR DIFFERANT"....NOW WAIT A MINUTE I SAID,..ITS NOT LIKE WE ALL HAVE ENOUGH GOING ON BEFORE SURGERY TO WORRY ABOUT THIS TOO.NO ONE EVER MENTION THIS TO ME BEFORE....SO NOW,THIS IS WHERE MY NEW FAMILY SHOULD BECOME ACTIVE,PAID EMPLOYEES OF THIS RESEARCH..IF THE SCIENTIST HIMSELF WAS A VICTIM OR FAMILY MEMBER,IM SURE HE WOULD HAVE THOUGHT OF THIS PROCESS..BUT WITHOUT THAT FAMILY INTERNAL LOVE AND BOND,YOU LET ANOTHER ONE GO BY."MAYBE WE WILL TEST OTHERS IN THE FUTURE THIS WAY "HE SAID,I HUNG UP WITH SO MUCH HURT,KNOWING THAT MY "HANK"WOULD HAVE MADE ALOT OF MY FAMILY HAPPY,BECAUSE WE WOULD HAVE TESTED FOR GROWTH,THEN TEST VERIOUS METHODS TO KILL "HANK"...

FROM WHAT I HAVE STUDIED,AND FELT MYSELF,THAT MOST OF MY BROTHERS AND SISTERS HAVE A FINAICIAL STRUGGLE AS WELL,ALL THE DOCTORS VISIT,MEDICINE,CAR TRIPS,AND FOOD..I THINK THAT MY FAMILY NEEDS TO BE GANEFULLY EMPLOYEED AT THESE RESEARCH CENTERS TO HELP OTHERS AS WELL,THEY HAVE THE DRIVE AND WILL,BECAUSE WHY?...THEY ARE FAMILY!!!!!!!!!!!!!

besides the medical problems that we go through as a family,like i said before the finacial problems that we have to be facef with is just as hard sometimes as our fight to cure the cancer.i know i said it before,but i mus stress my strong beliefs that those of the family could find a job within the research groups if all the research groups became more orginized,and generally located by type of cancer..i dont care if its 10,or one hundered of my brothres/sisters that secure a paying job at the centers,its better than not being able to work at all,and we all would benifit more from this because all these family members have a strong cause and will to think,and work harder for finding or assisting in finding a cause or cure for cancer,other then just collecting a hefty paycheck every two weeks,my family would feel alot better to collect anything awardable to be gainfully employeed,and helping in this cause..most of the victims end up losing thier jobs because of this cancer,due to time off,and doctors visits,its proven that most of them dont return back to thier past jobs..i often wonder now if employers look "down"on my family,thinking maybe we cant produce enough,or work hard enough?..well,let me tell you mr employer something..there are two big decisions that my family must think about..fear and hope...we will always have fear...unless you had your breast removed,your colin taken out,liver replacement,lung surgery,brain surgery,testicular surgery,and all the other forms of cancer related problems,..you will never never know what the word fear is..this type of fear is worst feeling that a person could go through..during this type of fear,it tends to take control of your body,and you have to fight hard against it.......

during the fear mode of our lives,we each go through a bit differant form of fear,and how we can deal with it...family and friends can be the best medicine for fear,being thier for you when you need them,and even when you think that you dont,they will be there..my fear came on me very hard..i was a big,tough,well built police officer for mchenry county county sheriffs police.up untill i found out about my tumor,i thought fear was pulling up on a call,and you see citizens running away from a house or apartment where somebody is firing a gun,and you run psat the citizens as they are fleeing,and your mind is telling you"wait a minute,if they are running away,why am i running in"?....it wasnt untill my brother kurt,who i love and admire so much,came to my home the morning after i found out about the tumor..it was here that i felt a differant type of fear,but yet so similiar in words..kurt,and my cousin bobby grabbed me,and kurt looked at me and said"come on scott,we will go into this together"..i felt no longer that i was running into that home by myself,but rather running into the home with a armored tank...it made me realize that yes,yes can deal with fear and go on.the night before this meeting with kurt and bobby,i had to keep reminding me that i have a lovely wife wendy of19years,and beutiful daughter jessica,and two great sons jon,and scotty jr...this night i had to take my service weapon aprt in as many peices as i could,i was shaking,but was afraid that i might do something that i shouldnt,just to be selfish of my pain and suffering..i was so relieved to know the true word of fear that next morning..it was a fear that i just had to deal with,.kept telling myself...the tumor is there,its reality,now just lets deal with it,it is what it is.

the second word that i talked about was hope...what is hope?..i found the definantion of hope by waking up in icu,and countng the how many cylinder bricks were there that made a wall..i knew that i made it out of surgery,even thou i wqas awake for about 9 hours of the surgery..hope was this new word that i had,but it wasnt a big word in emotion to me..but a couple weeks later i went to EVANSTON NORTHWESTERN HOSPITAL,EVANSTON IL TO SEE DR PALEOLOGOS.I walked into the waiting area with my wife wendy,my mother lorraine,and my brother kurt..i looked in the waiting area,and there approx 18 brothers/sisters sitting there waiting for verious treatments..some in wheel chairs,some using walking canes,some looked very tired and sick..but one thing stuck out from the beginning.they all would look at me,and or each other and smile..i didnt know anyone of these victims,nor do i think they knew each other,but those smiles as i smiled back to them made us a part of the family..we all knew and felt the unity that we would share..it didnt care that some of them were 15 years old,and others were in thier eighties..we didnt care or even think of us like that,we were that new family.

now looking back on the word hope,i took it for granted early on with my strugle.i have such a demanding and caring sister named karyn..as soon as i broke the news,or i should say wendy had to talk beacuse i caouldnt even get a word out of my mouth to mom when i found out about the tumor,karyn began to work hard on finding me a hospital and checking on my diagonise.karyn has her own home health care treatment business,so she has seen alot ot the similiar situations after surgery that i would soon to find out..but i knew with karyn working away at it,that i didnt have to worry about that end of it..i trusted in my sister,and she proved me right,time after time,...she replaced that word of fear with the word of hope..i made up my decision that right or wrong,i went with her advise and knew that i would never look down on it negative if anything did happen negative during surgery,she gave me hope,and where would i have been with out hope either?.a small country hospital by me that maybe had did one brain surgery in 5 years?.no,she knew what had to be done and how to do it..

yes my new family,i want you to meet your new mother lorraine,your new sister karyn,and new brother kurt..they dont have the diease that we have,but they are still your brothers and sisters,and will rejoice and me so thrilled to have such a big family..

hope doesnt have to be for those with cancer,no,its not limited to the family,but hope can be shared by all and help those with cancer,or any other disease or illness.all you have to do is join the family and help where ever you can...maybe be that 2nd policeman runnning into that house,or trying out your cooking skills,helping to sit down and find a solution to the fiancial problems,help with locating a job or place to work in the research area or any type of work,or simply take your brother and or sister out for a ride and show them something maybe they never saw before,..maybe a buffalo,a park,a new street,pizzari,any thing....help build that hope.

Preface

I don't know why, but almost every medical person that I have talked with doesn't know how we get various forms of cancer. Is it in the water we drink? Is it in the food we eat? Is it from a television set, microwave, a phone we use, caused from what we smoke? I mean come on, do you really even have a clue? I know that I am somewhat tough on scientists and doctors in the past for not finding a general cure, but I speak for all my brothers and sisters who I never had a chance to talk to, those who struggled for some many hard years—fighting every day to breathe—only then to leave us. They were firemen, football players, senators, business owners, fourth graders, and children in kindergarten. It doesn't matter who you are, how famous you are, or how much money you might have, you could be a part of My New Family.

So, it is here the reason why I am going to be such a tough SOB to all the scientists until they can stop this terrible illness, cancer. But don't worry, if you want to build a new style of car next year, they shall develop it. If you want more bytes or more RAM out of your computer, sure, they will develop it. Then, damn it; develop a cure finally for cancer, Mr. or Mrs. Scientist.

I won't stop hounding you, and I hope that My New Family supports me. It is not my war, but my family's war in locating the cure for cancer. Let me and my families assist you in finding a cure for cancer, but don't be offendedsive if we tell you how you might be able locate a possible cure. After all, we have this illness, and we have a stronger motive than you to get rid of it.

I have had conversations with several hundred cancer victims, and myself, they all tell me that, when first told of their cancer diagnosis, the next several days and weeks become a blur: trying to find out what it is, how to treat it, where to get treatment, and what the future is. I know that feeling. Like I had said earlier, I had my sister Karyn and brother Kurt to help me out in my time of need. I knew nothing at all about cancer and was clueless on how to get the treatments and fight it.

I wondered if my brother and sister and I can do this, why other brothers and sisters can't do the same for others. Also a good point to bring up is that from patient to patient the same cancer will be treated differently, depending on where you go for treatment. But if you were a broken car, and your causes for the break down were relayed to several auto dealers for repairs, mostly the same responses would be returned. Why? Because these dealers follow guidelines set forth from the auto makers. And the technicians who do the work on these cars are held to operating standards and reviewed often to insure a high level of customer satisfaction. Once the problem is identified with the vehicle, you should be able to go to ten different dealers and get the same—or close to the same—answers on how to repair your car. Sure, the only thing that would be different would be the price might be different from one to another.

Can you already see where I might be going with is? I know that every person is different. And using the broken down car example was meant only as form of comparison with something that we all use each day. We trust others' training and quality control and customer service to repair it, and we don't normally know how ourselves to fix it on our own. Cancer is cancer, and we now know from the millions of dollars spent on research that cancer is developed from abnormal cells within our body. Do we have an operating standard set forth for this type of break down? Do we have a quality control system in place for this? Do we have customer service? Yes we do, through several hundred different organizations that all differ from each other on how we develop this illness, how to correct it by treatments, not getting ten different types of treatments from ten different doctors, and of course the charges will all be different. Look how upset you are when you take your vehicle to the auto dealer for repairs, and it comes back less than one hundred percent. You would drive it right back and complain, wouldn't you? So I would get in my car, and drive it right back to the doctor and tell him to fix it, but then again, he might not know what is actually even broken. But perhaps he's just trying to get an eight-cylinder engine to run on four cylinders to get by. Isn't there a name that we call these types of technicians? Concentrate on what works to kill the cancer; don't hurt eight other family members and use them as test dummies for two other members. Hey Doc, what kind of car do you drive, and how many cylinders?

With my view on scientist, I know scientists have made great treatment methods for some types of cancer. These methods have assisted us in our living with our disease. I'm not blaming the scientists, but rather making the scientist aware that we are watching and monitoring their progress and want to find just one thing: the cure for cancer.

I have seen reports that say certain types of food you eat increase your chances of getting cancer or what you drink is bad as well. But then the following week, maybe on the local news they say drinking coffee or tea is good for your health.

There seem to be different views and studies on the same thing. One is good, yet one is bad. This goes back to my previous discussion about how scientists are isolated and working on different cures for different types of cancers. On making it more of a geographic scale of isolating the scientist who can work on one form of cancer, and yet have another scientist work on another cure for cancer. How many different scientists across the country for example are working on finding a cure for breast cancer? Any rough guess on the number? OK, let's make it easier for you to answer, how many in just one given state then?

I think that you might have picked up on my feelings by now as to how we, as a country, are doing to find a cure for cancer.

While I sit back and try to imagine how many different forms of cancer are out there, let me explain what I have learned about them.

Breast cancer is probably the number one form of cancer in females. It can affect you at any age, but statically I have been told that it is more likely affects you when are forty and, and as you get older. As with any form of cancer, breast cancer may affect someone a lot younger then forty. I strongly believe that women should have yearly mammograms even if they are feeling great, and healthy. Now don't go writing me a thousand letters yet, ladies, and telling me where I can go. Hear me out.

The American Cancer Society recommends that females in their twenties and thirties should have a clinical breast exam (CBE) as a part of a periodic health exam, preferably at least every three years. And it suggests that women over forty years old have it every year. If you have any family history, genetic tendency, or past breast cancer, then you should discuss this with your doctor and make sure he is aware of this.

I have talked to several of my new sisters who are—or were going through—breast cancer. Throughout this book, I will try to speak of a few of these sisters. If you are reading this book and the thought has ever crossed your mind that you might need an exam, please don't wait. My thoughts for your health don't end with only breast cancer, but several other forms that you need to be checked for. Colorectal cancer, also called colon cancer, endometrial cancer, ovarian cancer, cervical cancer, skin cancer, and lung cancer are all forms of cancer that you sisters could get. Early detection and awareness of the warning signs play an enormous role in correcting the illness and in formulating your treatment options. Knowing the types of cancer and how to detect them can make the difference between life and death. I don't mean to say that to scare you into treatment, but rather to show you that you have options. You can't leave your options up to just the doctors. I'm not going to sit here and speak badly about doctors,

xxxii   My New Family

but I feel that I must tell you that, if I would have continued to listen to my own doctor before my discovery of cancer, that I probably would not be able to sit here and type each day. I might discuss this issue about that Doctor later in this book, but probably wont because I want to save it for a trial date against him.

One last thing on this issue of breast cancer for now, ladies is that you should not even think about how a guy might react to you going through breast cancer or the surgical procedures. It's not there for him, (meaning your body) but you are there for him. If he doesn't respect this or is not supportive of this, tell him to hit the road. Don't even waste any time thinking about him, or how he might feel from the effects. Only worry about how to get you better, that's it. Shake my hand on this one, ladies. OK, now you can send me that letter.

And my brothers, this same bit of knowledge applies to you also. Early detection: listen to your bodies and let the doctors know what is wrong.

Prostate and colon cancers seem to be the leading. culprits with the male form of cancer. Again, with early detection, proper dieting, and exercise, the outcome risks can be lowered. As I have just spoken of our sisters who might be going through breast cancer and the loss of something they might think is so personal to them, I'm sure that you don't think of them any differently because of their tragedy, do you? Before you decide to think about that question for too long, let me put it in a different prospective.

Testicular cancer affects hundred of thousands of us. I really don't feel that the ladies sit back and actually think of how bad it would be to spend time or think of us wrongly badly of us because we might lose a few personal parts. But, guys, don't send me your letters yet. Give me one moment to explain this.

I recently have met two different ladies who both had surgery to remove their breasts. After a discussion on their outcomes and the battle they suffered through, I can honestly say that I didn't think one negative thought toward their personal loss. So I hope they didn't feel uncomfortable with it, just as you won't. You talk about chemistry in a relationship that makes it work for a lifetime? My guess is that someone with breast cancer and someone with testicular cancer would make lifetime partners and enjoy life much better then a female with 36 D breasts and a male with a fourteen-inch penis.

Let me have those letters, guys, and tell me if I am correct. And if not, you're missing out on something very important in life. Call it *chemistry*.

Now that you have got me on the topic of chemistry, let me tell you briefly about something.

Some twenty years ago, I stood at the altar and said my vows. Because of my brain cancer, I can't really recall too many details. But strangely enough, I can recall the vows I spoke. I had met this beautiful and caring lady named Wendy. I knew from the start that we had the chemistry needed to make our relationship work. My family believed in me, although some of Wendy's family didn't. I think that they only looked at me as perhaps someone that might just want to get to know her and then leave. Actually, it was totally the opposite. I didn't want to win over anyone, that's for sure. I did know that this girl would be the only one for me in my life, no matter what would happen. I thought I would be the one there to make her strong when she was sick; we could grow old and gray together. Society had tested our strengths and weakness a few times. I grew up from a weaker financial background then her, but it didn't bother her. At times, it seemed that she grew only stronger and stronger with my side of the family. Wendy would always acknowledge that I was the strong one in our relationship that kept things going. Wendy was tested by this thought thou just weeks ago when I discovered brain cancer and underwent surgery. Wendy was always there at my side, knowing just when I was feeling too much pain and giving me pain killers, or a better cure for my pain, a kiss. She slept next to me in the hospital and reached over to squeeze my leg from time to time. Here I had thought that I would be put into a position sometime in my life to help and take care of Wendy medically. I knew that I would be there for her 110 percent and keep her on her feet. Well, honey, I guess that it was your turn first to take care of me, and congratulations on a job well done. Each day that I wake up, I can see you look at me quickly, as if you are shocked or something. But I know you are just trying to check on my condition. In one night, you had to give up your job and take on a new role as my caregiver. In case I haven't told you today, honey, I love you and thank you.

They tell me now that I must prepare myself mentally and physically for a long battle with this illness. Physically I think I am OK. I will speak of it probably several times in this book, but I love to run. Running takes my bad blood and replaces it with my good blood. Yeah, I'm sure that medically this doesn't happen, but to me mentally it does. My body feels better afterward. You don't have to run thirty miles each day. Start out by walking and gradually build up. Check with you doctor first, and he or she should be able to get you started on a great routine. Other than running, I am not sure how else to prepare myself for this battle.

I know that the chemotherapy treatments coming up will be brutal to me. So what? At least I will be given this tool to use in my defense. Or I should say my offense? I will be the one crossing that scrimmage line, trying to pick up that extra yard (day), on my way to the end of the field to score a touchdown (victory over cancer). In this game, it doesn't matter if one or both of your knees are down. You may still be allowed to crawl—even after you are tackled—to gain that extra yard. Keep those legs moving! If you have to, crawl on your stomach for that first down, but just keep going.

You might hear the referee blow his whistle. I, as a youth baseball coach, must listen and respect the referee decision when he blows his whistle and ends a play. But in this case ignore the referee, and don't stop until you get to the other side of that field for the score.

My first game is against a team called Chemo. I will start with home-field advantage, first down, and only ten yards to go. My New Family will be my offensive guards, right and left tackles, center, and running back. I know I can at least pick up the first down.

Dear Mr. Senator

I remember growing up when my older brother, John, worked for a Chicago-area congressman part time. I had asked John at that time what a congressman does. John, with a straight face, stared at me for a few seconds then smiled and said that they are there to help you. He told me they were the go-between for the average person and the White House. I thought, "Wow, kind of like a big mail-man."

I never thought of that particular conversation with John during the past some twenty years, as John was taken by the Lord from a long-battled illness. It was just recently that John's conversation came so clearly into my mind. It was during the times that I had e-mailed my new brothers Rob, Bill, Buddy, and Nelson. It was while I was communicating back and forth with these new brothers that the meaning of John's discussion hit me. Rob was speaking for his own brother, Jose, who was recently diagnosed with brain cancer and was very ill. Jose was unable to communicate, and Rob was to be his go-between, like John said a congressman was for the public. I know that senators and congressmen work on getting things passed. They work on grants and all that nice stuff for us, but wait—can't you, Mr. Senator, take on a few more duties, just for us, the American public, let's see if its part of your job duties?

Now being a senator, you have to be elected to the title and office by us, the American people., and the voters. If a bit of John's conservation was true when he told it to me, then you are the one we need.

Each district is represented by one of you, Mr. or Mrs. Senator. We will divide each state into districts also (the same districts as yours) and have a brother and sister of My New Family working with you. You will take on at least one of the family members. It will be part of your duty to set up a database within your district for those of us who have cancer and volunteer to be involved in this database. Each district shall have at least one MY NEW Family member working with you to help prepare such a database. This database will not simply be names of cancer victims; this database shall contain up-to-date research findings and tests for cancer cures.

For example, Brother Matt calls you about his throat cancer. You should be able to retrieve data on this illness, including support groups, medical facilities, and other related helpful information. We are not asking you to become a doctor, but rather to be our go-between person. We are not asking that you must refer one doctor over another doctor or determine which doctor is better then each other in your words or opinion, but to simply be able to reply and say, "OK, this is what's available to you. Here is the research about this type of cancer, and the doctors and medical facilities that treat it."

A senator's office should have up-to-date telephone and e-mail contact information and progress reports for treatments and cures for cancer.

The Internet, library, and other sources of information on these topics are full but often out-of-date at times. But you, Mr. Senator, should have the most up-to-date information. Remember, you are that "big mailman" that John talked about years ago. When a family member finds out that they or someone else has cancer, they should be able to go to their local senator's office and review the documentation. If not, then maybe we have the wrong go-between person. How hard is it for us to punch a different hole in the voting ballot then?

For all My New Family members, this could help you get back into doing things by helping your local senator make this information available to everyone. And if not, I'm sure we all know how to get our local senator's phone number. So, Mr. Senator, you now have a strong reason to watch the progress of curing cancer a bit stronger, and if not, I hope your ears can hear good enough then, I would like then I'll to be the first to call you!

My Monday Checkups

It's now Monday morning, and the first thing that I do is send an e-mail to my brothers and sisters to see how their weekend was and what this week brings upon them.

Usually there are doctor's visits and treatments to take care of. But that's not the main reason for this e-mail. The main reason is to comfort them with the fact that they have made it through the past week, and they can still use that wonderful word "*hope*". I type to Jose, who can't read my e-mail; his brother, Rob, reads it to him. Jose has brain cancer, which I have been told has spread throughout his head. Rob tells me the doctors are trying to help him, but other doctors say there is nothing they can do for him. Jose walked into the hospital, just like me, and was runner in good physical shape, also like I was. Now Jose can't walk without assistance. Yes, it is a big, very big change for Jose, but he still holds onto that hope, and I can tell that he smiles when we send e-mails or joke back and forth. I always love to joke around; that's one thing in my life that I have excelled in, as well being a caring person. I give Jose some referral names and phone numbers of my doctors to see if there is anything that they can do medically for him. I know that I help Jose each day just by giving him moral support and comfort.

Next I type to my new sister Carolyn, who is fighting breast cancer. Carolyn has both fear and no hope pounding on her mind daily she writes to me.

I try and comfort her and tell her to let the fear subside and let the hope take over. She tells me that she feels better by e-mailing me, even though I am her new brother and a man, and that she has reduced her fear by talking to me about something so personal in her life. Breast cancer is a very touchy subject for my sister Carolyn, probably for any female. I realize this, and I have to be careful on this subject, as talking about female body parts has always got me in the doghouse with my wife in the past. Somehow I always lose in this type of conversation with my wife, so I know I must be very careful. The doghouse nowadays is way too small to fit me (OK, maybe I'm a bit overweight), so here goes my reply:

"Carolyn, I am sorry, but it's your mind that controls your life, my sister, not the place where your cancer is located. Some of my brothers have lost parts of their body that they had once thought was their mind, but weren't!"
"Carolyn, you are not in this alone. Couldn't you help someone else going through an early stage of cancer by talking to them, like I have with you?"

Carolyn didn't hesitate and replied: "Of course I will."

I hoped I was able to avoid the doghouse with Carolyn; she sounds like a truly wonderful lady who can help other people as well. I referred her to others who have breast, brain, colon, and other forms of cancer. I did not limit my referrals to those who only had breast cancer, since now she understood our goal as a family. Now she was eagerly on her way to help those new family members now!

My "good morning" e-mails, as I call them, get sent to so many of My New Family members whom I have met either on the computer or the phone during my battle with brain cancer. The list is piling up now in numbers it includes friends, neighbors, fellow workers, and strangers who I have just spoken to for the first time.

From the very first day I found out about my brain cancer, people would often tell me, "Please, if there is anything I could do, just let me know."

I replied by saying, "Thank you. I need nothing from you right now, but soon I will come to you and ask you for a favor."

Almost everyone whom I said this to was cancer-free, and very few of them had family members with cancer. These wonderful people had no idea at all that soon they would become a part of My New Family. Some would become members not by choice but rather by having a form of cancer themselves, and the remaining would become members as brothers and sisters for support or technical issues. Like I had spoken of earlier, s

Support services could mean that you send an e-mail to someone with cancer, send out a get-well card, cook a family meal one night for them, and or just make a quick phone call and say, "Hey, I just wanted to call and say hi." In your brother's or sister's eyes, that could mean the difference between night and day—the feelings that someone cares. Or let's say you stop by to see your sister who has been ill with cancer, and you take her for a ride to the new Target store that just opened up and walk around and buy something. More importantly, you have just spent some time with her, other than at a doctor's office. Share a cup of tea or coffee, and this day would feel like a new beginning for her, and hopefully for you as well. You have the power to take a bit of fear and replace it with hope. And then hope will continue to grow within her.

These are just a few examples that I have used myself in my support service role, but there is a technical role as well. Some of you have this technical role, you could be an accountant and maybe help family members with their financial issues, or maybe a mortgage loan broker could lower their monthly payments. These are what I call technical type jobs that people work each day, and could share a bit of their time by helping others out. There are those of you who could help out with finding medical treatments and care options, like my sister Karyn has done. But I guarantee you that if you harm my brother or sister and try to take advantage of them in any way because of their weakness in the illness; I will come after you with everything I have. My New Family members will join together with me to make sure you are found and punished.

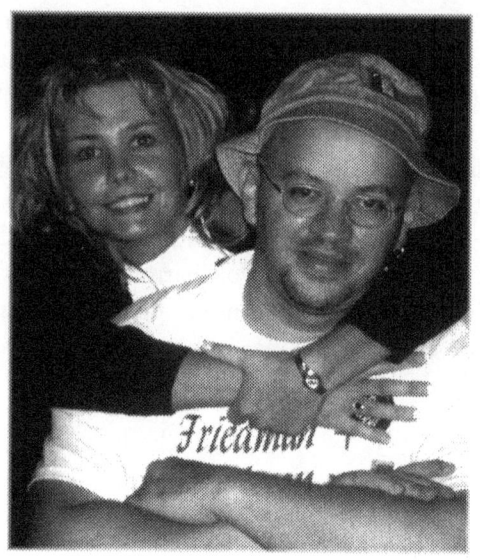

Buddy and Kim

Membership

I'm sure that our members consist of a wide variety of walks of life; there are gas station clerks, restaurant workers, fireman, policeman, lawyers, accountants, and just about every type of worker that one could imagine. All these members can help by donating a little bit of time. And having cancer doesn't give us the right to take advantage of those whom are willing to help us; neither, we should be held to the high standards as well. These wonderful people who help us out will be doing so from their own hearts, and we should always realize that what they do for us is their way of joining our family. By their choice, not by causation.

I don't care if you live in the south side of Chicago, Miami, Burbank, or Tacoma; it makes no difference. Like it or not, we are all one and the same family. We are part of one large family. We are members of My New Family. We think of each other on all holidays and celebrations, such as Christmas, Hanukkah, or any other religious event. Think of it for one second, what a large kick-ass family we would have, huh? We can work closely with the organizations that are out there providing information and support on cancer issues.

Well, it is now night fall, and I must send my good night message to make sure everyone got through the day OK, assign them some homework to do for the week, and sign off until the morning. Good night.

As I make my rounds on the Internet to check on my family members, I think about how the past few weeks have been much more positive for me. Several of my brothers have shown good progress, and they have spoken of doing daily things now, trying to improve each day. This makes me feel like a camp counselor, going around at night and making sure each person is in their cabin, lights off, and prepared for the next day. Tonight—October 15, 2002—is also very difficult for me, as my brother Buddy from West Virginia was feeling down a bit, and rightfully so.

Buddy and his wife, Kim, were very instrumental to me from the start, for it was here on my computer that I first found my friend Buddy, just one day after returning home from my brain surgery at the hospital.

We continued to send e-mails back and forth, and soon became best friends, although I have never met my friend in person yet. We sent pictures of each other back and forth and quickly added these pictures to our own family picture album. We were both proud to place the pictures in the album and show them to everyone. Yes, a long-lost brother, one might say. Tonight, though, Buddy was admitted back into the hospital because of complications with his previous brain surgery to remove cancer. Buddy tonight is in a lot of pain, but Kim reassures me that she is talking with the doctors at the hospital to lower his pain level. Kim is one tough sister, always making the doctor's appointments and keeping good care of Buddy. Kim has been assigned a new role in her life; she is now a caregiver.

I feel so hurt tonight, knowing that my brother is back in the hospital. I can't wait until he gets back home, and we can play again. Maybe me and Buddy against Billy in football?. I know that tomorrow will bring better news from Buddy. I have no doubt.

I have been trying to reach another brother, Mark, for almost eight weeks now, with no reply. I have finally just received a reply from Mark, and he states that he was just released from the hospital after having a hemorrhage and further tumor removal. Mark says that he had lost feeling in his left arm and left leg and told me, "Hey, but I still held on to the power to send e-mails to ya, though."

I sent him my reply, thanking him for being so strong while we were away from each other for those weeks and asking him when we can run together again. We both love to run. We live thousand miles apart, but we both agreed that we would run and leave cancer in last place then!

Tonight I will sleep with one eye open in case my brothers need to talk to me.

After sleeping for more than ten hours tonight, I still find that I'm tired. It must be from the thinking and prayers that I ask for each night for my brothers and sisters before I fall asleep, so being a bit tired feeling is well worth it for me. Buddy's son, Noah, will chat with me on the computer and inform me of how his week was. We would talk about school, reading assignments, new games, and tease each other about girls. Noah gets a big kick out of reading my simple jokes that I send him (yes, all clean jokes, he is ten years old).

I tell not only Noah, but my own children, how I find reading books brings me a relief from pain. As you could probably see by this picture of me, any comfort from the pain is a comfort. This is what my children must wake up every morning to see, before they go to school. Its not like I can hide this or anything either, as wearing a hat or anything could increase the odds of catching a infection. Also, I am confined to this hospital type chair in my living room until I get better, which I hope comes within days. Jessica, Jon, and Scotty, sorry you had to see this, but you know that I went under surgery to show you all that no matter how difficult things might look in life, that giving up is not a option. We are strong kids, we can and will make it through this obstacle in life, together, as well with My New Family.

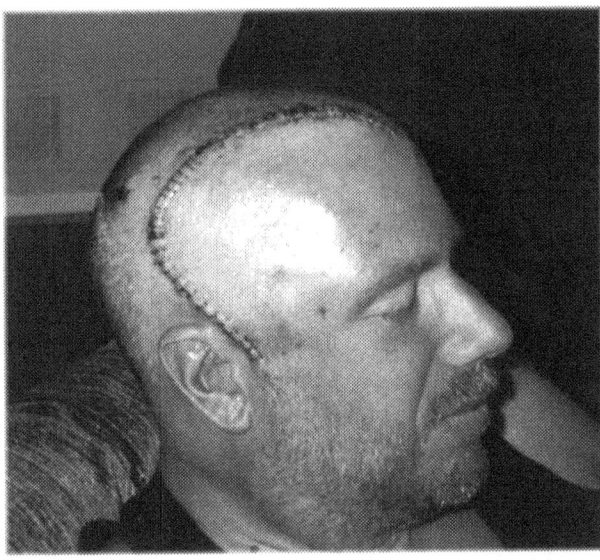

Author Scott Milliman

So now that I am awake, I begin my roll call. Turning on the computer seems like I'm turning on this huge machine filled with my whole family within it. I know that by re-reading my last sentence, it might not sound correct, but read it again. I hope you see and feel what I feel each morning then. I tell my brothers and sisters good morning, and to get out there and suck up some fresh air, and to build willpower and hope today. I have just hung up the phone after speaking with Buddy in the hospital. Buddy seems very tired and worn out, but he sounds upbeat after talking with me for a few minutes. I warned him that I had better not find out from any source that he is lying there in the bed watching those afternoon soap operas shows that my wife enjoys watching. I tell Buddy that it's OK to watch the nurses walk down the hall from time to time though, and if he needs a partner to help watch, then to call me. We both break out into a laugh together so hard that I think I better slow down or I might hurt my little brother.

Buddy reports that once he feels better the doctors will be able to transfer him to Duke University hospital in North Carolina, which is where he had the original brain surgery. He seems very happy about this news, so I am as well then.

After speaking to Buddy, I review my next brother's e-mail. It's from Bill in Wisconsin. Bill reports that he had his first round of radiation treatment now and reports on how scared he is, but he states that he feels so much better after we talked together. I tell him that it's OK to be afraid. It's natural, but hopefully the fear level will lower. I tell him to bring that hope level up and to stay positive and strong. Bill agrees with me, and I give him my oncologist's, Dr Nina Paleologos from Evanston Northwestern health care, who I feel is such a expert in brain cancer research, phone number for a second opinion in his case. Bill later in the afternoon he sends me an e-mail that reads, "I walked outside today, looked up, and tried to soak up as much of the air and sun I can, and I felt good also."

This was a nice reply. I kept a handful of my own outdoor grass shavings with me. When I went into surgery, I had a full pocket of my yard grass; I wanted that smell and feeling to remain with me. Although several people questioned then, and maybe even now, my mental status of thinking because of this, but unless you are placed in a similar situation, I'm not sure you can understand the simple meaning of having a handful of your own lawn grass with you, or looking straight up and soaking as much air into you as you can. I still recall the male nurse placing me on my stretcher and pushing me toward the operating room that morning. He asked me while pushing, if I had anything on me, like metal objects or anything at all, and I simply replied, "Nope, just a pocket full of grass."

The stretcher came to an abrupt stop, and he said, "Grass, what you talking about? Did you smoke that shit this morning? We are going to brain surgery now; we can't do that."

I simply laughed and said, "No, grass shaving from my yard. I picked a handful and wanted to keep it close to me."

The look he gave me made me laugh even harder than before. He thought I had really lost it. I told him that I had planted the grass from seeds, watered it, cut it when needed, and walked on it when I needed to, and the grass always kept me supported, never letting me fall.

So now you know that to make something grow, you must care for it, water it, cut it, and more in order to show that you want it to blossom and be a part of you. This is the meaning of My New Family. I never cared if the grass was yellow or green; I still treated it the same way, just as I do now with my brothers and sisters.

How many of us actually take the time to realize every morning, that another day is here? Do we realize that there is a heaven upon us and over us? I enjoy the feeling on my face as I grin. That grin is made up of two parts: one part skin and one part life. The skin, into the mixtures a given. It's up to you all out there to show up and bring the life" Part of life" to complete the ingredients or the smile or grin.

The second part is simple people. Just smile. Just by you being a part of someone's day, you can bring life to them. And you know what? By doing this, you will be able to complete several orders. You would be able to serve more that just one person., I'm sure it would.

Consider yourself as a chef.

A few people have asked me if I believe in angels. Yes, I do. It might not be the same as people traditionally think of, though. I don't see wings on their backs, but at this point. I do see wonderful angels each day. I see them in you, him, her, or them. I see a part of an angel in all of us. We all have it.

No, I wished at times that I was crazy, but, no, I'm not. Look around at all of us. There is truly this image in every one of us, every day, in each city, each street, or road. Maybe society just doesn't recognize this, but just sit back and think about it for a moment. Remember when you may have said or did something that would cause someone to laugh? Remember when you may have done something to help someone, even if you never met the person before? Was it maybe a phone call, or saying hi to someone at the store? Maybe it was the way you smiled or shook someone's hand? Well, for the sick, we see this Angel among us that we just described.

I still can't get over my previous writing that spoke of how I think our local senator might be able to help in this battle. If I can help people across the country, don't you think a senator could help out even more in just his district? in large amounts, since the area will be smaller and isolated by districts? I am not looking for eight hours a day or even two hours a day, but rather minutes of time to make a difference in a child or adult's life. You, Mr. Senator, could be holding the source of information for a mother who is reaching out for to help her child. I surely would hope that you wouldn't even think about slapping that hand reaching out, would you, Mr. Senator?

Do you happen to know how many hands you might be slapping by just slapping that one hand? That one hand is connected to thousands of other hands; do I have to say more, Mr. Senator?

Yesterday I took my fourteen-year-old son, Jon, to a local Sear's eye center, in attempt to get his first set of contact lenses. Jon, like anyone else would be, was a bit scared about having someone touching near his eyes for the first time. This day was very difficult for Jon. Sears employee Maria met us. Jon felt confident with Maria, so I sat off to the side while she tried to show him how to place the contact lens in his eyes. We arrived at 3:50 PM, and Jon tried and tried to get the lens in and out. Jon was getting upset with himself because he really wanted the process to go smoothly, but nerves would take over just as his finger touched his eye and he would blink, causing the lens to fall. I tried to give Jon words of encouragement. Maria kept up with Jon, talking and trying to get this process completed. I heard Jon tell Maria how badly he wanted to play football at his high school, and tonight was his first practice. He couldn't play unless he had the contacts in. Now we all know what happens when we want something done, and time is ticking away. The pressure piles on you then. I then heard Jon tell Maria, "My dad will be so proud of me tonight."

There was something special about Maria, the way that she handled this whole situation so tenderly, but there was something else that I couldn't figure it out at first.

She never gave up on Jon.

She continued to work with Jon, building his confidence, even though he was getting more upset because the lens would not simply just get into the eye. Then about at 6 PM, Jon finally got the contact in, and he had one big smile. Maria grabbed the cordless store phone and called her mother to pick up her children from school, since she said she would be late tonight. I had no idea that the store closed at 5 PM, almost one hour before. She told her mother that she was doing some special training.

Jon was now able to put the contact in and take it out. He stood up and gave me a big high-five. I thanked Maria and had a short conversation with her. It was here that she told me that her husband, Tom, had recently been killed in a vehicle accident just blocks from her home. She observed my large scar on top of my head and asked me about it. After a brief explanation, she stated that her best friend's daughter, who was only a year old, had been just diagnosed with a brain tumor, and that the parents were so confused about where to go or what to do.

Now this all kind of came together, the time that Maria gave above and beyond at Sears tonight, her not giving up on Jon, and my realization that I was a part of her best friend's family—My New Family—and would try to help them, just like Maria did tonight. It is strange how you might meet another new family member, isn't it?

Am I for You as You Are for Me?

As you continue to read my book, you should see that My New Family can develop and branch off in the future to help others in need. There are a few programs that I have been trying to test, and so far the response has been only positive. Am I saying this book shall bring world peace? Am I saying that this book should bring you to better mental and physical condition? I sure hope so! I hope that this book is not only read by cancer victims but by those who have any type of illness. This book is about giving and receiving. It is up to you to determine which one you do, or if you do both.

I can't even count how many times someone has come up to me and expressed how something like this illness can happen to such a nice person. My only thought of a reply is that someone a lot higher than me wanted me to have this, so that I might be able to help not one, but thousands of others. I am up to the challenge. I will begin to lift weights and run again. I will start back slowly, but at least start up again. I am not a quitter, nor do I want any of you to be. I wake up feeling sick the same as you do. I feel the pain and discomforts like you, and I feel drained and beat up at times just like you do, but let's keep pushing. Get up and do something. Don't let the illness and treatments dictate our response to cancer; let us dictate our own response.

You should be able to bring some hope and a better feeling about yourself on your own. Our new brothers and sisters can help us pick each other up at times and get to the next level. Live life now like you never have before; it could be better then it was five or ten years ago. Sure, maybe we think that certain times in the past were the best ever, maybe that vacation cruise, or spring break, or our own wedding. What ever it might have been. Still retain that beautiful image, but work on getting better now, and, when something comes up in the future, you will be able to taste and enjoy it better then. You have already tasted life once before, but now, wait until you live it better by adding your own spices to it, it is going to taste so much better. If it would have meant I lost my leg, then so be it, but get out of my way; I can still walk on the other leg.

As I continue in my writing of this book, I wonder why and how people get cancer, and how long it has been around. I can see that one of the most important factors for fighting cancer is early detection. The earlier the growth is detected, the better chance we might have for victory. There is now a lot of focus on early detection of breast cancer for my sisters through self-exams and mammography testing. We still lose approximately 40,000 sisters each year to this form of cancer alone. I praise the organizations out there that are helping to fund breast cancer research and prevention. It is really starting to get recognized now, but only after losing so many sisters in the past years. So, my sisters, I beg you to take at least one day a year, put it aside, and use it for a checkup, which might include a clinical breast examination and routine mammogram. I don't care if you are feeling fine and just got done completing a twenty-five-mile marathon; you must go once a year. I have talked to sisters who really didn't want to get the one-day checkup, but they would make sure that their carpets in the home were cleaned once a year and having the oil changed in their car twice a year. Why should you be any different?

In the year 2005, experts estimated there would be 200,000 new cases of breast cancer. My sisters, you must assist yourself and do a monthly self-exam, and just because you might feel something, maybe like a lump, don't freak out and think the worst, and stop there. Follow up with the doctors right away. Experts report that eighty percent of lumps are not cancerous. That tells me that at least eighty percent of my sisters are now taking proper medical follow-ups then. You go, girls; you can make a big difference, one at a time. And for those who find your lump non-cancerous, you can help another sister who has not had such good news yet or is still waiting for test results.

I must admit that it's a bit hard or awkward for a brother to discuss a personal issue so personal to my sisters as like breast cancer. I look at it as cancer. I don't care what type you have, or where it is located in your body; you both have it, and what I try to seek is proper guidance and support. That is why it is so important that our senator's office should contain the most up-to-date booklets and research on every form of cancer. I have read some great literature out there from organizations fighting cancer, and I honor those groups. Everyone should have the same option to read the same great booklets, but most don't know where to look, and the Internet is just too filled and jammed with information—some good, some bad—and what you choose to believe could result in a life-or-death decision.

Let me tell you what I mean. If you go there right now, visit six different hospitals or doctor's offices, you might see three or four, or possibly even five, different local and national organizations' booklets lying out on the waiting tables for people to read about cancer. Some of them will be about the same form of cancer but with different ideas and approaches, and of course with this come different attack strategies to fight cancer. Horseshit, I say. We, as brothers and sisters, have long been used as guinea pigs for the programs to battle cancer. Enough is enough!

Just as it might be hard for me to talk about my sisters' breast cancer, we must address my brothers' personal side of cancer, testicular cancer. Guys, if you feel a lump, or something else that that maybe shouldn't be there, go to the doctor and have it checked out. You heard me speak to the ladies about losing something so personal to them, and just like you we can be put into that same feeling. So it's not about being "Macho" for us, or looking like a model for her, it's about living. Just ask your doctor on one of the many self examinations out there for all of us to do, and we should always follow through with the doctor visits, and testing as recommended for early detection. It's not macho to be sitting in any type of surgery, get my point across? If you need to feel more macho thou, go ahead and send me a complaint letter. I will add it to my stack!!

The talk of cancer doesn't have to always be negative. I have learned during my short passage here on Earth that sometimes, if you think or talk negatively about something long enough, that it will eventually become negative. In general, someone talking about cancer will be sad, negative, angry, and so forth Try this reply.

The next time someone you meet asks, "How are you?" Simply reply, "Good. And you?" Call it a deflection of some sort, or whatever you want, but I see it as a positive motivator for yourself. Here, try it again.

"How are you?"

"Good. And you?" (I heard that.)

So you see, if you can make yourself feel positive, then be positive. While we are on this topic, I would like to share with you a few pictures of people I have met who kept me positive. Some of them have cancer and others don't. I am not going to tell you which ones have it. But they have one thing in common: their smiles and positive attitudes. Most of these pictures were taken either on the day I discovered my cancer or close to it.

Get yourself a fresh hot cup of Gloria Jean tea, coffee, or your favorite drink, and let these wonderful people enter your life, like they have done for me. I have also included portions of e-mails that I receive each day for your reading. Some are from Australia, Turkey, Greece, India, and many other countries, along with ones from almost every state in the United States.

Jun 19
"Okay Scott, I feel so much better! You're awesome, for the first time I feel a little consoled".
Georgia

May 7
"Good to hear from you. I'M on Chemo and it makes me tired, but other than that I can't complain. Any plans for the summer?"
Florida

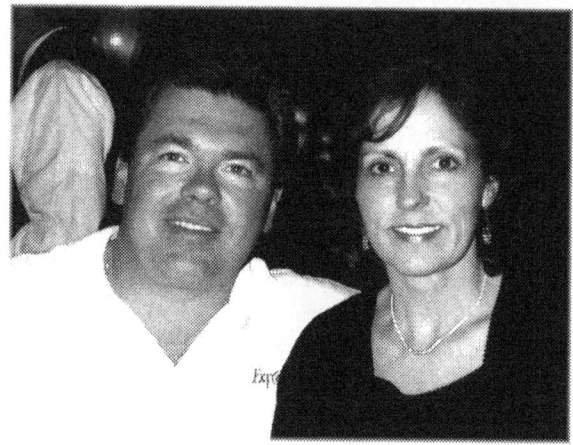

May 14
"Just wanted to tell you thanks for all your thoughts and prayers. Its one year at this point from when they took the tumor out. Wow!"
Wisconsin

March 15
"this is Jennifer's husband, Jim. I would love to talk to talk to you; my typing skills are not the best."
New Lenox, IL

June 18
"My son is nine years old, and just had cancer surgery. It is not an option for us to lose him."
Vancouver

June 1
"Scott, so glad we met, thanks again for taking the time out of your busy day to speak with me. We need more people in this world like you…"

Louisiana

May 21
"Scott, I'm sorry, but he died this morning at 3:45 CDT, sorry."
California
(This e-mail above was sent by the father of the man I have been talking with.)

June 27
"Scott, Lee, and I think you have been such an inspiration to us, thank you for caring."
Anita

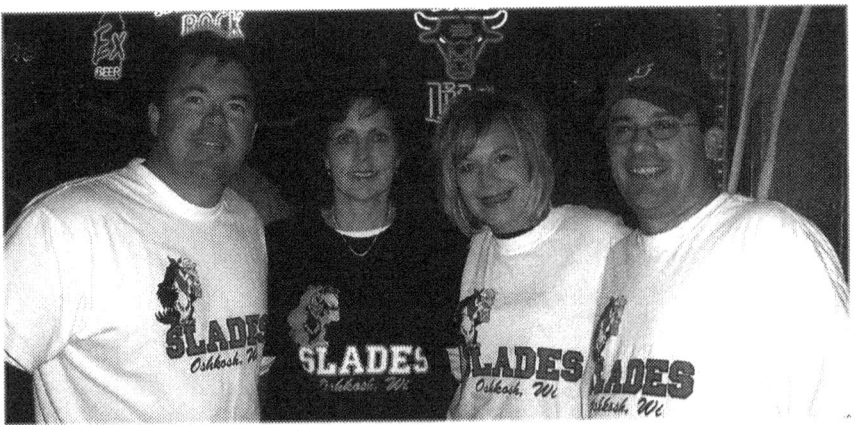

September 5
"Scott thanks for the e-mail".
Cleveland

November 27
"Jen is coming home tomorrow; she has to learn to walk again."
James

October 18
"I got your e-mail, and we all are fighting the same battle. It's been scary for all of us."
San Francisco

September 5
"Thanks for your email. What type of cancer did you have?"
Indiana

August 14
"I came down with phenomena and pleurisy, so now I'm dealing with this. I hope that all went OK with your best friend? As far as being scared, yes I'm still very scared. Thanks."
From me.

November 11
"Going on week twenty-two tomorrow of chemo. Hope we can get through this for many years."
Wisconsin

November 27
"I know he loves talking with you every night!" Florida

September 10
"My mother is an eighty-five-year-old survivor! She is living proof that we can survive."
North Dakota

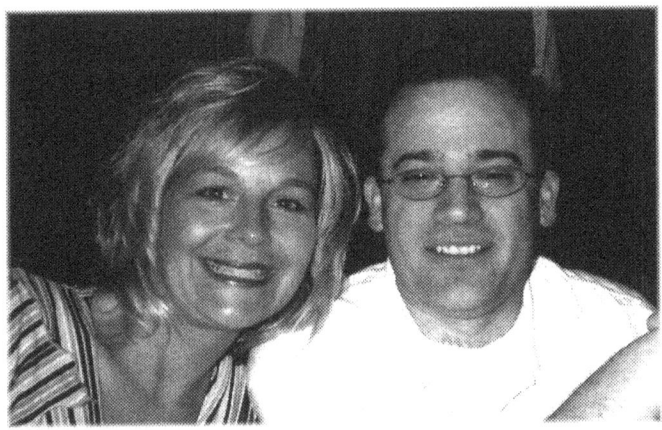

October 29
"Scott, be positive and hopeful, and find out all you can about current treatments. Our son, also named Scott, lived nineteen years with the tumor, and worked most of the time before he died."
Peter & Sandy
(Thank you Peter and Sandy)

October 16
"Hi Scott, yes I like to run. I used to run half-mile marathons, 10 Ks, I'm going to start back walking and work my way up to jogging, then running."
Marc
(Sorry you didn't get that chance, Marc. Watch over us please.)

February 15
"Last two days didn't go so well, I got constipated from all the antiit-nausia med's that I'm taking."
Texas

October 26
"Scott, thank you for your prayers for my brother Jose. Unfortunately, he passed away last night. Thank you for your compassion and empathy."
New York

March 4
"Boy, you sound like a "man on a mission." Great, I agree there should be a centralized site for cancertreating scientist to find the cure!"
Florida

January 20

"Very good to hear from you. My brother goes home tomorrow. He has been in rehab. I mentioned you to him, but wasn't very responsive."
Oregon
(NOW ME AND HER BROTHER KYLE TALK ALL THE TIME, IT'S GREAT!)

Oct 15
"Sorry it has taken so long to get back to you. I have been in UCLA Center. I lost control of my left side due to a hemorrhage, hope you are doing better."
California

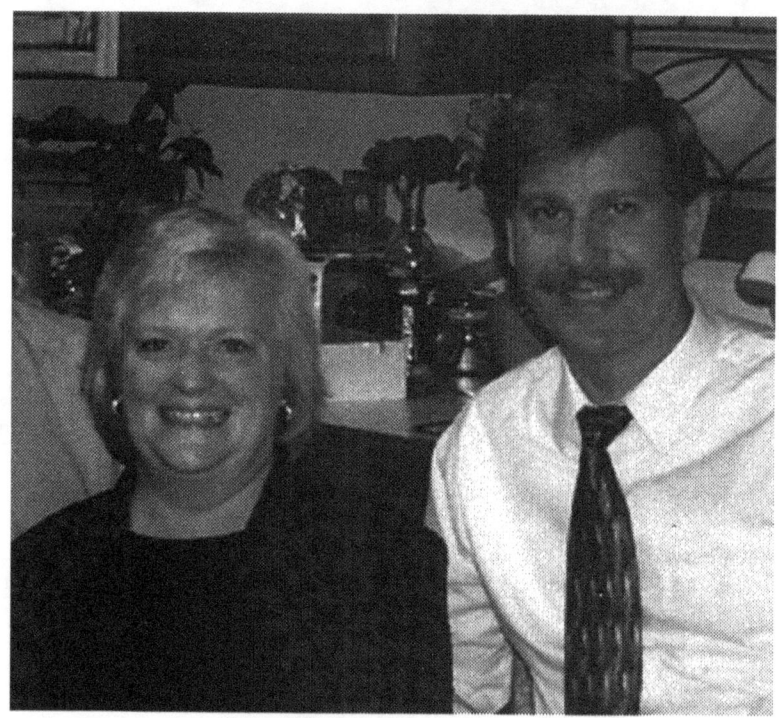

Dec 31
"Scott, my wife Jenn passed away. Jenn was my friend, my soul mate, and wife. Keep fighting, Scott, and do not give up. Oh yes, keep emailing me!"
James.

Mar 17
"You mean a lot to all of us, you have been a lifeline for Buddy & Kim, and I want you to know how much I appreciate it and thank you for it. Have you ever heard that "FRIENDS ARE YOUR CHOSEN FAMILY??" All my heart you are like family to all of us, and I know he loves talking with you every night."
North Carolina

Jan 2
"You bring up some very interesting points, it makes me stop and think things I take for granted every day. I know that there is nothing that I say to change things, I'm loss for words, but I figure the best thing that I can do is be there when you want to talk, or get you out of the house once in a while."
Mike Lucas
Illinois
(THANK YOU MIKE…you have just spoken about My New Family. Welcome aboard my friend.)
Scott

Oct 21
"What an amazing story, Scott. You and I have a whole lot in common."
Texas

July 26
"Would you mind emailing a friend of mine who is a retired police detective? He was diagnosed four years ago. I'm sure it would be good for him to talk to you and tap into your amazing strength. Please let me know if it is okay with you."
New York
(Of course I will…another great example of how my membership works.)
Scott.

Dec 12
"I miss him very much. I'd give anything for one more day with him. Emily misses him very much too. She keeps asking when she will see him again, and why he had to die."
Washington.

September 8

"Hi Scott, I have the same exact type of tumor as you and in the same spot. I had brain surgery two months ago. Can you tell me about the chemo that you're on? Thanks, it helps ease my mind a little. If you could get back to me when you get a chance, I would appreciate it."
New Jersey

April 11
"Dear Scott, Hi, I hope you don't mind me adding, but I would like to tell you how much we appreciate you writing my daughter. If only you knew how much happier she is when she gets a reply from you. It really makes a difference to her. So, that is all I wanted to say., again thank you for making such a big difference to our little girl's recovery. Thank you for being her best medication, especially when you have your own health to worry about."
Australia

June 19
"Sorry I have not been in touch.-y You are a wonderful correspondent,—always so upbeat. I myself have some lengthy medical problems, but each day that I get to e-mail with you, I feel much more comfort in life."
Cornwall, England

June 22
"Hi Scott, sorry to bother you, but I need your help. You have a friend that is experiencing the same visual problems as a friend of mine and I was wondering if you could connect the two of them so they can discuss it. It would make a world of difference for him."
Oregon.
(Connection from Oregon to Madison, Wisconsin)

As I go further in my writing of this book, I sometimes feel as though as if I were in a wind tunnel, bringing people to me. That is one of the reasons I wrote this book, to bring people with and without cancer together as one family. I must say that I was initially shocked—I mean sickened—by some of the statistics that I discovered about cancer victims. According to the American Cancer Society, 555,000 Americans are expected to die this year from cancer alone. That is 555,000 brothers, sisters, husbands, wives, children, grandparents, friends, workers; the list of names goes on. This figure should hit you like running straight into a freight train. It's very real. Half a million of us. Terrible.

How many of us pass away because there is not enough (or incorrect) knowledge and treatment of cancer? I don't know. How many have passed away because they all shared one thing in common: cancer? My guess is 555,000 sisters and brothers.

Children as they grow need to become a part of My New Family from an early age, not hopefully from having cancer, but rather by learning from what might and might not cause it. They should be taught proper nutrition and exercise and chemicals and pesticides to stay away from. Since helping one brother feels so good, could you imagine how you would feel if you helped hundreds or thousands of people in your lifetime? You have the power to start with helping one now. Go and begin.

America has gone through a lot of tough situations in the recently past, such as terrorism, which continues to hurt and change the way we as Americans live each day,. By the threat of terrorism But were these changes as devastating to human life as cancer has been to my family? I am not trying to take away any sorrow or pain from the terrible attacks on September 11 that we all felt, but nothing can even compete with the loss of 555, 000 brothers and sisters each year. No cruel, evil leader can take credit for this. But cancer could, and it did. Cancer is truly among us all, and we must fight back and start winning this war. Join and enlist with My New Family, and be proud to take it on and fight it.

Another day light begins. And it's a Monday morning. I can only pray and hope that all my family will be there to answer my e-mails. I know the news has not been good for my brothers Jose and Buddy lately, but I never give up hope, and I shall never show them any weakness. I continue to try and make them laugh with stupid jokes. at times. The original jokes, though, were sent to me from a fellow worker from who is a firefighter for Park Ridge, Illinois. He allowed me the chance to forward these to my brothers and sisters, and some of the jokes would make one cry from laughter. At the time I was given the credit for these nights of jokes and laughter, but it was you, Buzz, who made these nights happier. Thank you, Buzz, for being a part of My New Family, and don't stop caring.

Buzz, I loved the paragraph that you told me, on how I should make greeting cards and such, while I was home now for extra money.

Lets see, you told me about the card to give to a ex-wife,which read "when we were together,

You said you'd die for me,

Now we've broken up,

I think its time

To keep your promise.

Then there was the one,

"your friends and I wanted to

to do something really special

for you, for your birthday,

so we're having you put to sleep".

And for my brother Buddy out there in West Va

'HAPPY BIRTHDAY UNCLE DAD!

and then there was the one on welcoming a baby into

this world

"How could two people as beautiful as you,

have such an ugly baby?

I'm glad that I went with my gut feelings, and stayed to becoming an author Buzz, rather then a card shop owner.

Here's a joke for you. She is so blonde, that she sent me a fax yesterday, and put a stamp on it.

Jose, although you may lie motionless I am told now, I hope that you can pull a little more life into you so you can get stronger. Buddy, I am told, is still having severe headaches and not feeling well overall. I know that the talk now of having a third brain surgery to remove more tumor growth scares you, and it makes me nervous as well, but I will be there for you again, waiting for you to chat again on the computer or the phone. In the meantime I continue to talk with Buddy in the hospital, and we agree that if he has to go through the surgery again, that I would have to eat something called buttermilk pie. I didn't like the name of this pie from the get-go, but I'm committed either way. Kim, who is Buddy's wife, must go home and play Mr. and Mrs. Mom to their two small children after spending all day with Buddy in the hospital.

OK, I admit that I have goose bumps now, not because of Buddy going through the surgery, I know he will do just fine, but knowing that I'm going to eat this buttermilk pie.

Now, midweek, I look back on the last few days. All my new brothers and sisters have made it through their struggles yet another week. Keep going, guys. Push, don't give up.

I don't know about all My New Family members, but for myself I have tried for the last several years to be careful about what I eat. I am an avid exerciser and love to run and run—sometimes more than twenty-five miles a week.

It is in my belief that "Sixty percent of all cancers are curable by means of lifestyles, like smoking, sun exposure, and poor diet."

I myself don't smoke, rarely go out in the sun, and am not one for a poor diet. OK, so I guess I'm in the forty percent table that is left out of the study? As for the doctors, they say that they don't have no idea how I got my cancer. I do know that there are more than three million people helping to conquer cancer. That number is fantastic. Great, I said, hurry. But should I ask the question now?

No, I don't think that each one of you know what I was going to ask, but it might not be fair to all those hard-working people, who dedicate sometime their own time to help, and for this I thank you and know that your actions will help all of us. If I ask you to explain the term *cancer*, what it is exactly, could you explain it at all?

Cancer is defined as an uncontrolled abnormal growth of cells, and these cells are responsible for causing more than one hundred different types of cancer in various locations in the body.

Come on now, you mean to tell me that it has taken several hundred years to try and find a cure for abnormal cell growth? I mean, it's not like you haven't had enough samples and trials available to you. You have more than 500,000 each year to review and examine. This means that by the time I have finished writing my book, each day trying to balance myself in the chair so as not to fall off, and trying to find the mental and physical ability to write, that we would have lost another 1,370 brothers and sisters. That would mean thousands of sisters losing their breasts, brothers losing their colons, children losing their chance of being juveniles, and what do we have to show for the past twelve months then? A better way to make gasoline, a new way to build automobiles, more ways for the wealthy to remove fat from their bodies so they can look younger, and of course some of the biggest breakthroughs that they are happy about is Botox and erectile function cures.

Ok, some more jokes. She is so blonde, that she tripped over the cordless phone.

Put some of this on the back burner, guys. Let it simmer while you cook up a hot recipe to cure this deadly illness for dinner. Guess who is coming to the first dinner? That's right. Mr. Senator will be the first dinner invitee. (The name "Mr. Senator" keeps popping up for some reason.)

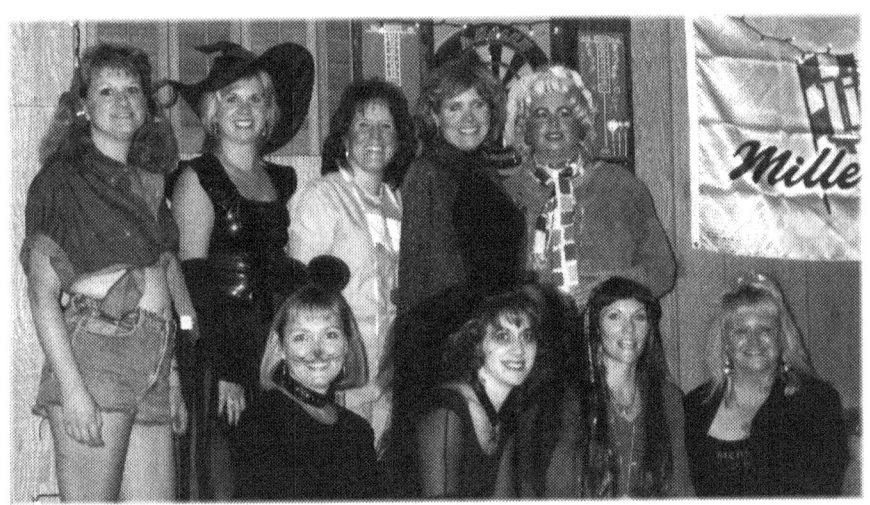

Time for Friends

This past Saturday night was a fun night for me and my wife Wendy. For the past several years, we have both looked forward to Halloween time. We meet our friends and have a costume party. The years go on, and the parties get smaller. It seems like everyone is being pulled in their own directions—between work, children, school, etc. We all are guilty of saying, "It's been too long, let's get together." But then a week turns into a month, and then into another year, and so on and so on. There are thousands of reasons why we allow this drifting apart to occur. Before my discovery of cancer, I attempted several times to go fishing, or just to meet for lunch with one of my good friends, Dave. He always blamed work as his reason for canceling our meetings. I am glad I tried to get us back together, though, and I am sure it will happen sometime soon.

Wendy and I went to this year's Halloween party. Dave was not there, but there were twenty-five or so of our friends there. Yeah, we talked about the recent brain surgery I had, and I drank my 7-Up while they all toasted each other to another year with beer and wine.

Next came the usual dart game we love to play. My friends laughed, spilled their beer, and held onto their stomachs from laughing pains as I threw my turn of darts, missing and striking the stringed lights that were hung for decoration, landing a few darts in the wall, and somehow missing the entire dart board. We all had a great time, danced, and hugged each other at the end of the night. We made plans for our annual Friday night fish fry the week before Christmas.

I wrote this past page to explain something. As we all said good-bye for the night, I could see each one look at me, and their eyes would fill up with tears. Each person did this and would ask what they could do for me. I then would reply there was nothing yet, but sometime soon. We looked at each other, smiled, laughed again a bit, and gave hugs and high-fives. As I walked outside in the very cold weather to the van, it was hard to believe that just ten weeks before I had gone through brain surgery. I had completed two full weeks of chemotherapy. I felt so good there tonight. Watching them all stand outside the door, waving at us as we drove away, brought more tears to my eyes.

Here it was Sunday morning, and I felt so good lying in bed, though I missed church, which I wasn't happy about. But I was still feeling so good from the Halloween party the night before.

This is what we all need sometimes, to enjoy a night with friends during our time of healing. The Monday morning after this, I received a phone call from the party host, who has been a close friend of ours for years.

She said, "Scott, I know you went through a lot, but I need your help."

I was thinking maybe her husband said something to offend her, or she had some other minor life problem this morning. Julie stated that her father had just been diagnosed with cancer, and that she and her family don't know what to do.

I calmed her down a bit and questioned where her father was and what type of cancer he had. She told me that it was a fatty bulge under his arm, which was already tested and found to be cancerous. I went to work right away, checking with other brothers out there who might have had this and doing some research. Julie wanted to know if just the local hospital was good enough to treat this form and if this type of cancer spreads elsewhere. I told her to contact an oncologist, who she then called. Julie cried and told me how thankful she was to have such wonderful big family, and that she classified me as her big brother.

Well, Julie, yes, we are one big family now. The word went out that we need to find a defense against this new battle with Julie's father. We all dug in our feet into the ground and got ready for this next fight; the incoming fighter planes had a name on the side of them: cancer. But we were going to win this battle.

I truly believe in the saying that each day is a new beginning. One would feel this expression a lot more when they are faced with life to life decisions. You have a new perspective for the water you drink and the food you taste. Most of the time food will taste different than before. Now you can actually feel the food hit your taste buds, then simply just floating right thru. I am now a bit more observant of what I might eat. Being on chemotherapy alters what you might have a taste for, or can hold down, and how you might feel. So at times you might not feel all that hot, but it's OK. The next day wake up and tell the cancer, "Today you are mine, sucker." I would go out and push just a bit more, and jog a mile and a half. Let the cancer know that you are fighting back. I don't care if you are lying in bed. Raise a leg or arm a few more times than usual; let it know you are in control. Just push a bit. I know it's hard, but just a little here and there adds up. One extra leg-lift here, one extra shoulder-shrug there. Do whatever you might think will work for you. It might be walking with a friend to suck up some sun outside, or even with that four-legged friend the dog, or simply raising your eyebrows a bit more today. Just don't give up. Remember, the little things that we might do are a plus for us and a negative for cancer.

I recently received a word finder book from a neighbor. After he left, I looked at it and remembered my grandma sitting there doing these puzzles in her home. I had a smile because I remember Grandma never quitting or giving up. I began to do a word puzzle finder today, and let me tell you that it was very difficult for me. The more I did, the better I felt. This process that I just went through was called my new beginning, as these word finders taught me a lot more about life than simply solving them. If I could solve the word puzzle, then I did something more today to help fight my battle with cancer.

Time for a joke again,

She is so blonde, that she wanted her friend to meet her at the corner of walk and don't walk.

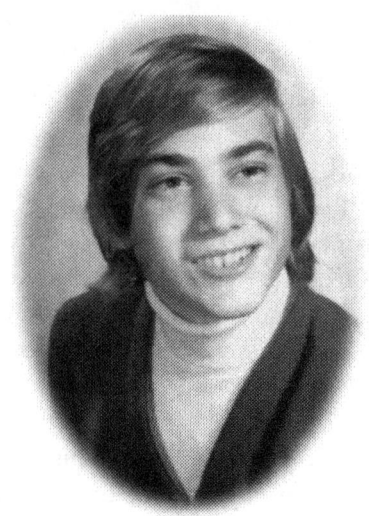

John

This next topic will be very difficult for me to type, but I will continue because I know that when this is done it will help not only myself but hopefully you as well. This was not prewritten or thought out before I begin to type, but rather I know inside me that I must type, and the words are going to come straight out. Here we go.

In my discussions with all My New Family members around the states, I found one thing that touches my heart so deeply. and that most people can't take thirty minutes out of their time to stop and pick up a friend or even a close family member who is suffering with cancer and take the person for a ride or even sit down and have a conversation with them. John, this is for you, my lovely brother.

My brother John was ill,(actual blood brother) confined to a wheelchair. I talked to John a lot on the phone, and when my busy work schedule allowed for free time, I would go over to John's home and chat. We were brothers, very close brothers. Sometimes these days were far apart, and we started to drift apart. At times I would think, or try and reason, that John's wife, Patti, or his best friend Kenny would be there on those days that I wasn't to take up the slack and chat with John.

There's no doubt John was so close to my heart. John helped me grow through high school after my father passed away. John was always there for me when I ran into a stumbling block of life. He never asked for anything payback at all. He was such a smart boy; he would try and help me in math and other topics of learning that I was weak in. More importantly, John would help me out with the best subject at all: that being life. Shortly after high school, I began work at a local suburban police department doing various jobs such as dispatching, record keeping, community service officer, and animal warden. I could always tell that John was very proud; he would always listen to the police scanner, and then quiz me on my language skills on the radio. Boy, John, you don't know how much that meant to me. And thank you Village of Wheeling for giving me this opportunity, and start in my life.

One busy night while I was working the midnight shift, John called me on the phone. We had a wonderful chat, although it was very busy that night with emergency calls coming in. I had to ask John if I could call him back.

"It's OK, Scott," he said. "I just wanted to talk to you. How about after you get off work at seven you come over for breakfast?" This would be 7 am, since I worked 11pm to 7 am shift, midnights.

I told him that sounded really good to me, and that I would do is run home, take a two-hour nap, then drive over there. John only lived about twenty minutes from me. We both said good-bye, and I went back to my busy work. Then at seven when I got off, I went home and laid down for a nap. About an hour later, I was awoken by my wife, saying I had an emergency phone call. I jumped up and thought I forgot something at work. But it was my sister Karyn on the phone, screaming that Johnny had passed away in his sleep during the night. I rushed over to John's house, but it was too late. The ambulance had left already, but the men and women of the Des Plaines Fire Department knew me and Johnny, and they couldn't bring Johnny back, although they tried. I completely lost everything that morning. I felt there would be nothing left for me, my heart and head hurt so bad. This is my brother, one that I played with each day growing up. One that made me what I am today. One that I will forever miss, and wished I could have it all back. Just for one more hug, one more, one more to teach me how to change a tire, one more to go to the movies, one more to listen to the crackling of that police radio John, and wait for you to call me and tell me if I did it right, or what I need to do and change. One more I Love You Big Brother.

"Johnny had diabetes," I cried, "how could he be gone because of this?" I cried? First my father passing away because of this, and now Johnny?...no. I could not accept this.

For the past eighteen years John, I have been trying so hard to figure out what you wanted to say that night, my dear brother. I'm sorry that it took so long to figure it out, John, but I know now. You wanted that ride in the car. You wanted that thirty-minute chat with me. You wanted that hot dog from the local burger stand right around the corner from you, didn't you? But mainly, you wanted me as a brother to be a part of your life, which contained your illness, and help you as well.

John, as a policeman, all those foot chases and domestic calls that I went on and handled, having to put my life on the line for others, never really felt like that much of a threat to me. I always endured the few beatings that I was involved in because someone didn't like the police, or someone hitting me with a barbeque grill over a domestic dispute. No problem, I would get back up and continue. I must do the same now, and realize that just because we have cancer, and may be down and weak, it doesn't mean that we must continue to be down. We can get back up and fight and I will John. Now, as I face my battle with brain cancer, the thing that sticks out the most about this whole ordeal is that I knew I always had the love and care for others. Sure, I was a good neighbor, a good father, but lacking in one thing, I didn't have that little "extra," as I called it, to take that extra step and help others more. It has been with me all these years, though. John, I like helping children, participating in the Shop with Cop program for Christmas shopping with cops and kids in need. I also enjoy shoveling my neighbor's sidewalk. If I'm already out there, I just keep continuing. But there were so many more important things that I was missing out on life, like helping those who really need the help more, and that's why you have given me the strength and willpower to put these whole feelings into work. It has already helped countless people across the country—all my daily contacts that I try to guide in the right direction to seek out the best in medical treatment, medicines, and to listen to the word that John was trying to tell me that night.

Hope and Care

Now that I know the direction of my life intentions which is to help others in need, I feel as though I can wrap my arms around each one of you, like we are all in a big circle like we used to play in grammar school. I bet that if you think hard enough, you could probably recall seeing that circle when you were in school, and maybe recall a few faces of children that you might have held hands with. While you were forming that large circle and holding hands, it gave you special feelings, I'm sure. It gave you a sense of comfort and happiness then, knowing you were close to someone, and making each other smile. This same feeling is what I want to engrave in you now, as you go and help your members of My New Family. How long in time spent, did it actually take by holding hands during that recess in school yard, and forming that circle to make you feel good? It was only minutes of time. I'm sure that it wasn't like half the day sitting out there, although it felt like it was.

Some of us would have tired out and left the circle to go play something else, like kickball maybe. Kickball, huh? At this point in my life, I like to call kickball as *work*. When you are tired of holding hands and feeling good, off to kickball we go. Out of the two games played, didn't holding hands make you feel better about yourself? So, that circle can be sending e-mails to brothers or sisters then. With all the fancy, high-speed Internet stuff, sending e-mails takes a fraction of the time than it would be via the circle. And heck, you can send get-well cards on the Internet now. So now one can enjoy the feelings of the circle, while still playing kickball. You can make more people feel better in those ten minutes of time than you can ever imagine. So come on, hold my hand, and join the circle, and make a difference! Playing kickball meant that you must kick something for a distance. Kind of the same when a kid is at the school grounds, and two teams line up and play kick ball, remember how this played,or do I have to explain yet further in detail on how to play kickball in school?

Ok, good, I was getting tired of that anyways. Ok, so kickball is kicking something. Now, we can still hold hands like in that circle I talked about right? And we can play kickball by kicking this cancer out of our bodies, or help others do it. Now you understand what I was trying to say, no?

Another joke. My wife doesn't watch football to much, because she is blonde, and thought a quarterback was a refund we can get.

As I sit and look out the windows of my den, the weather has been changing to the type of season I love best: fall, then winter. It is the holiday time, the changing of the colors on the leaves, the cloudy days, and the cooler temperatures. Holidays always bring good feelings to me. I don't know what the weather's like in the rest of the country today. While thinking about this, I receive an e-mail from Robert in Florida, who I never spoke to before. Robert explains that he was referred to me via another family member. Robert doesn't say much in his first e-mail to me, other than asking me if I can help him. I reply, and ask Robert what might be wrong (I suspect maybe cancer). Robert replies back to me later that evening and says he doesn't have cancer, but still needs a huge favor. OK, we are starting off on the right foot then. I'm glad to hear he doesn't have cancer. There is something obviously bothering him, though, and his next several e-mails are short, but I can tell there is something there. Robert tells me that he is thirteen years old, a healthy little guy living in central Florida. Robert overheard his mother talking on the phone with a relative, crying, saying that she had breast cancer.

Robert asks that we all pray for his mother, and, "Doesn't breast cancer for sure you mean you die?"

I try to comfort Robert a bit, and reply, "No, my little brother, it doesn't mean that at all."

I tell him that it's important she continues seeing her doctor and follow treatments. Robert says that his mother is not seeing a doctor and said she doesn't want to either. I tell Robert that I will reply back to him within just a few hours. I need to see what is out there in Florida. I contact a sister who I previously spoke to named Shawnee, who also went through breast cancer treatments and lives in Florida as well. I tell her about the e-mail that I just received from Robert. Shawnee calls me back at my home within thirty minutes and gives me the phone numbers for Y-ME National Breast Cancer Organization, along with its e-mail address. I forward this to Robert and tell him that his mother can feel free to contact Shawnee or myself if she likes. Robert says he will call right away and replies, "Cool, maybe now I can go to school knowing Mom will get help."

What such a big responsibility for that little guy. I did speak to Robert's mom late the next day. I told her about possible financial aid from the State of Florida, after she tells me that her employer had fired her after twenty-three years. She tells me that she suffered from memory loss—basically from birth she said. She reports that it never really affected her growing up much, and there hasn't really been a question at work at all about her ability to perform at her skills, but that her boss felt that she has become a possible liability.

Dear Mr Boss

"What?" I ask. "This is stupid. I am surely going to write this Mr. Boss."

She really doesn't want me to use her first name much, she feels so embarrassed she says. She feels confident talking with Shawnee, and that makes me feel better. I think that I need to ask our brothers and sisters to write Mr. Boss letters and maybe some of his vendors that he works with. I know next time I take my family to Walt Disney World in Florida; my first stop will be to see Mr. Boss. Hey, Mr. Boss, have a change of heart yet? Well, it has only been four days since I talked with Robert's mom, and I have received two phone calls from Mr. Boss in central Florida. I try to decide if I should call him now or wait. I'm not a bad person, so I return his call. He begins to tell me that he is unaware of how serious her condition was, with having breast cancer now. Robert's mom had got herself so worked up over the past several weeks, worried so much, that she could hardly remember her phone number. There was too much on her mind at once. What I intended to be a peaceful conversation, led to me yelling at him for even thinking about letting her go, because she has breast cancer? I mean, come on, what's your thinking you idiot, I tell him. I guess at this point our conversation was over for now. I don't think that I even had time to boil the water, for a Gloria Jean Tea time, the phone rings again. Mr. Boss tells me that he wants to help out so badly, and advises that he will get the proper forms and help file them for her disability claim to help the family.

"Bingo," I think, "he just said the key word, *family*."

Yep, I wonder if he has any idea about My New Family. He doesn't, but he was sure beginning to feel the heat from it. He tells me that he hopes she gets the best treatment, and after recovery he wants her to immediately come back to work for him, but in the meantime, he wants to make sure her children are taken care of. It's been a short period of time since I heard from her or Robert. I have been told that she had a double breast removal, and is beginning treatment, including chemotherapy. Shawnee reports that Mr. Boss has given her and her family money for her time off, plus six extra weeks until the disability benefits kick in. I ask Shawnee if she could have Robert e-mail me when he can so that I might say hi. I did get the e-mail from Robert, who tells me that it's still very scary, but he has a lot of people coming over to check on him and his mom. He asks if I can come down there next week to visit them. No, my little brother, I can't next week, because of my medical treatments, but maybe next summer I will be better enough to travel, but here is a picture of me until then.

Robert's reply comes back later after seeing my police academy graduation picture. "Wow, how can that big of a guy be so nice? You look like you should be a big mean guy, like the Terminator."

Does Robert mean my physical size, or my inner size?

Lack of Communication

Over the years watching and listening to television, some talk shows discuss why sometimes one person feels one thing, and yet another person may act or feel differently on the same topic. Experts say it's from lack of communication. What does this mean? I guess maybe it means not talking enough to your wife, spouse, or children or listening to their input on life. It is interesting to me, as I recall back on these statements made about that, and I often wonder maybe if we all just have that explanation out of tune." a bit. Lack of communication means just that, the failure to communicate. So why was that book about guys being from Mars and women from Venus such an eye-opening experience for some people? Because it showed how one person thinks differently from another. OK, that's actually a good theory. I'm sure it helped a lot of people. But my definition of lack of communication is the failure of a person, people, or group to identify a problem among others and act on it.

Could this mean the failure to stop at a stop sign or the lack of attention that you might give someone? I still think it's from failure to identify the notification; the notification is your ability to help others, like My New Family. This notification the warnings about cancer have been passed down to us time and time again, but most people feel they can get through life without the fear or concern of cancer affecting them or a close relative. This is my definition of lack of communication in my words. You can go on and on, thinking you are OK, but then it hits home. Then you begin to scramble around trying to find information on cancer, trying to find doctors, financial aid, and all the other items including surgery that will be on your dinner plate real soon facing you. And guess what, now you have just become a member of our family. Member of the new family. I was, no doubt, one of those in the past that who did not realize the meaning of *lack of communication*. As you read from my past, I paid a very hefty price with John for not learning this before. I know for a fact, that it just didn't take me getting brain cancer to realize this, though. I would always help out from here to here, helping others, but obviously the wrong people. I helped politicians get elected to office. I helped them put up signs and went door-to-door. Then I would race off to work.

I helped the wrong people in life. I'm not knocking our political leaders, but rather stating that I should have spent that time taking a brother for a ride, calling a sister on the phone, and taking a little guy in the squad car to see what it's like to turn on the lights and siren.

I'm sorry to those who should have been a part of my life and weren't. I believe that no one is to blame, though. Most of us had the chance to grow up like Billy, or Suzanne as children, living every day to play. Yes, those were the great days, running out into that field, waiting for a baseball to be hit to you, or dressing up and going to a tea party at Susan's home. But if there hadn't been a Billy or Susan, where would we be then? All those growing pains, all the different relationships, all the different schools. Looking back now, Billy and Susan had a tough time growing up, and often looked to others for guidance and direction. It might have come from their father, mother, brother, teachers, or neighbors. Didn't most of these feel like your family already, Billy? This is when Billy should have been taught how to help others in the family—the family that is not just limited to relatives. Cancer affects at least one out of every four people now, maybe even more. Teach them at an early age on how to communicate with My New Family, and yes, yes, yes, there will be plenty of time left over to catch the ball out there, or have that tea party.

For a portion of this book, I have spoken for those of My New Family members who are unable to speak right now. My New Family members continue to spend their day trying to find the best care they can or trying to come to grips with their news. If I had a candle in my home for each one of you I have helped, without taking self award for achievement, I would never need light bulbs in my home again. The flame from each candle would glow so brightly and oh so proudly. I just recently saw that a Hollywood movie star was diagnosed with a form of brain cancer. The articles all said that fellow movie stars were trying to find him the best help. I'm sure money was not an issue for this person, but how about my poor brother who works sixty hours a week doing cement work? Yes, Mr. Movie Star, I do feel for you and your family. I'm not making light of the situation here. I will pray for you, and also Sammy, my cement worker brother. I don't want to even hear the argument that "Sammy chose his profession," because he probably didn't have a choice. And He made the best of it. I just want the both of you to get great treatments, get cured, and then communicate maybe with each other on about your new brotherhood. You both are stars in my eyes, and both of you should give out autographs.

The e-mails I received today talk mostly about progress and are positive at that. "I continue to push," one writes. Some speak of walking outside today, and others tell me they are handling the chemotherapy a bit better this week. Hey, that's great news. Most have begun to push the fear out of them, and replace it with more hope. Hope is not guaranteed to make you live fifty more years, but then again it could. Those of you who are still in the hospital today, thank those who print our e-mails and read them to you. If it means that you have been able to keep our eyes open a bit more today with less pain, that's great news. Don't give up.

I just reviewed a recent e-mail from you, Linda. What a way to start, "Do you know what it's like having a breast squeezed so hard and then cut open? How would you like your balls to go through this?"

Oh my gosh, Linda, you are a sister to me. No, I do not know what that feeling is like, but I feel for you, my dear. I look at the e-mail address, and it is the same as Robert's, so I think Linda must be Robert's mom. Now I feel that we can move on with my writings, now that I have explained my version on lack of communication. It is now Sunday morning again, and I begin to review my e-mails. On Sunday, I love to send out my e-mails with a lot of faith behind them. I continue to pray for all My New Family members who made it through another week. Does it mean that if God chose to take a brother or sister that he was not listening to my prayers? No, not at all, and this was proved to me each day during my reading of e-mails.

Today I received two new sisters, one with ovarian cancer and the other with breast cancer. They both seek for a simple friendship to help them as they go through their battle with cancer, exchanging words of encouragement, hope, faith, and will. I ask today if either has been given support information groups or referrals. Both advised me that they have been referred to a list of agencies, but that the list is too long and confusing., to confusing the sisters tell me. One of the girls advised me that the list is "not clear, no real path to follow." she reports. I tell her that knowledge is the best, to get the most knowledge she can on her cancer and the treatments available, and I simply suggest that she contact national formed organizations like the American Cancer Society and Y-ME. No, these sisters won't get any information from their Mr. Senator yet. I have called and left messages with various federal officials on this topic, and all said, "Let me take your name and number, and I will have someone call you." I will keep typing, rather then sit and wait for a phone call from them. So far, no returned phone calls.

So Long, My Friend

I scroll down my e-mails and open one from New York, one that I hate to read. Our brother Jose has been taken away, it says, no longer fighting the cancer. Lord, I know you heard every one of my prayers. And, yes, I know you were listening. Just please take care of all the other family members who are still fighting this, and pray for Jose's family to bring comfort. I guess this was like that saying, "For every door closed, a window shall be open." Jose, thanks for your hard fight, for being my new brother, and I will continue to help others. Be good to us and watch over us, Jose, and help us too. No, Jose, you didn't lose that fight. Sure, it gets harder on some Monday mornings to sit here and type after hearing of such loss of one of My New Family members. I ask the family of the lost brothers or sisters if I can continue to keep them in my e-mail address book and include them in my week. Everyone replies without even thinking twice, "Of course, we are still family members!"

Every other week I would get the same question from a brother or sister, "How can I help more?" Well, the most important thing you can do is not give up, keep fighting, stay strong, and keep positive. Other than that, I'm sure that the new family members who don't have cancer but are a big part of My New Family wouldn't mind at all if you help them out: send an e-mail, give someone a call, or check on someone. Sister Janet Weech tells me often that every day as she drives through the country on her way to work she observes the large corn fields, and this helps her to relax and pray while driving for not only me but others with cancer.

As each of us feel better and also for those who already beat cancer, let's locate our local senator, write down his name, address, and the phone number for his office. It doesn't matter if Mr. Senator is a Republican or Democrat; they both should, and are going to, share an equal demand from us. It will take one My New Family member—sister or brother—per district to represent us to Mr. or Mrs. Senator. If we have five, twenty, or thirty or more family members in each district ready to represent us, that's even better. The more people who help and make sure that we all get the latest information on cancer, the better. It sure would be nice if we could get at least one brother and one sister to represent us per district. I feel confident this could get accomplished without much struggle. I think the title of district captain would be an appropriate title. Each district captain would be briefed by a state spokesperson. Again, this will be a joint assistance forming of one female and one male at least, and the addition of a child less than eighteen years of age would be encouraged to represent the voice of our youth. I will speak more about this idea in a further chapter.

I have just read in a very popular American news magazine that the federal government is thrilled" to have an organized plan on how to control the grouping of organic foods. This is set up to make sure proper labeling is done and allows the purchaser to be more aware of what they are actually purchasing. The article also stated that after a several year battle," the guidelines were finally met. I laughed after reading this article. I continued to read the whole magazine in an attempt to find anything else of value to the average American. Yes, there was an article about the terrible sniper attacks that put so many people on guard in several states. That was really a nightmare for several hundred folks. I felt sorry for them. In further reading of the magazine, I couldn't find one article on any form of cancer, but did congratulate the federal government on the findings on organic foods. Do you know how I feel about all this right about now? You bet I was very disturbed. I thought that I would check the past several issues in case I missed something. Nope, same old thing: discussions about issues overseas and how or why we reacted to the terrorism in our country. It hurts all of us when innocent lives are taken; there is no reason for that either.

As a country, we lose more brothers and sisters to cancer than anything else. Over a half of million of us—yes us—each year. There should be a very high priority each day to find a cure for cancer. What should this top priority task force be named, then? How about the Jose, Julie, Rebecca, Liz, Phil team? I can name the lost brothers and sisters as long as you would like me to. Just pull up a chair, and I will continue naming them for days, and from my heart.

How many of you sit around with family and friends on New Year's Eve and enjoy the few hours together, a few drinks maybe, and make your New Year's resolutions? Was it to go on a diet, stop smoking, to change jobs? These are all very good resolutions. Hopefully you made these important changes and carry them over until the next New Year's Eve party. I do know sitting there this New Year's Eve night, I would have already made my resolutions many months before, and the number one was to fight this brain cancer aggressively, and my second also came several months before, being a person in a position to help others with cancer. This position has not limited me to just being able to be home more, now that I have less to do, but rather the ability and drive to want to help others in a time of need, during their battle with cancer. This position is not only held by me, but all of you. This is about you being in that same position to help others.

Don't you feel good when you go to church, shake the hand of someone you never met before, and say hi to them? This reaching out of your hand to someone else is the same when you shake your hands with to a new family member. Some of my friends surprised me. While I did not ask them to, they sent e-mails to Jose's family yesterday, giving them words of comfort. The making of new brothers and sisters just occurred again. You gave me a good feeling, guys! My dream of bringing people together and helping others was just further accomplished, but sad to say it was through the passing of a brother. The new brothers and sisters control their own willingness to help others out now in the future.By doing this, it should make you feel stronger, healthier, and happier.

One particular sister replied to me about how good she felt, and that this has made her the happiest she's ever been, just by spending fifteen minutes a day. She also replied that for the past seventeen years now, she has been making New Year's resolutions to stop drinking. She is an alcoholic, and no treatment made her realize life more then this fifteen minutes a day sharing with someone else a email or saying hi to someone. She also reports that though being an alcoholic is not as bad as having cancer, she can't help either herself or others if not alive, and, "I can't give up the booze, but I sure can help out in life. "She replied

What a wonderful e-mail. Although alcoholism is very serious, she downplays it for others with cancer. I hope that she will one day beat her illness as well. She asked that I don't use her name in this writings because she has been unsuccessful in her attempts to get off alcohol and is on probation. She was afraid I might tell the police department. Tell the police department what, my sister? That there is a sister out there who is trying to help herself through others and is trying so hard in life. That's what I would say!

Loneliness is the one feeling that most people have that I have talked to about having cancer. In all actuality, we are far from lonely. We have the largest grouping of common illness in the country, then anything else. But for some reason, living with cancer for some reason makes us feel that we have something wrong with us. We often want to hide the fact that we have it, and have a hard time telling someone that we have this "c-word" illness. We worry that others might look at us differently, as though the cancer would jump out and attack someone who might be talking to us. It is not some weird illness that developed overnight, causing us to grow a third or fourth arm and glowing bright green color. Come on, we have cancer, a common illness. It's not brought on by some space Martian or something. We are humans, the same as you are.

When you get sick from the common cold or flu, you might have to change your eating and sleeping patterns a bit, don't you? Well, sometimes we must do the same, depending on how we feel with the illness or the effects of the treatments. So tell me, where are we different then? We are different because we, who go through cancer, join a large family together, and taste life in a different way. We know what it was like to take our bodies and ourselves for granted. We now enjoy the taste of our food, the air that we breathe, the feeling of grass on our feet, having of tea time (peace time) just for ourselves every day, the love for family and friends, walking the dog, or working forty hours a week. We do all these things because we can; we have cancer.

Today is yet another Friday, and again I look back upon my week. I'm getting ready for my business, side job, whatever you might call it, but I'm getting ready for Monday already. Most would probably think, "You are crazy. Here it is Friday, and you are getting prepared for Monday's work. I mean there are still Friday night fish fries, a little bit of clubbing, hanging out with friends and family for the weekend before Monday strikes again."

Over this weekend someone might need a little bit more encouragement, or someone might get admitted to the hospital on Sunday for Monday morning treatments or surgery. Who knows, this might be a double e-mail weekend for me. Yes, this is my Friday, my business, and I most spend a few minutes to prepare for the next work week. Sure, I might spend some time this weekend on the business as well, but it would be less time than most people would take to read the newspaper. For me, this is time well spent. My business is My New Family.

Maybe it's still hard for you to realize the effects cancer might have. I am now looking at an e-mail I just received, guess from which sister this came from?

Thanks, Linda

'This past weekend has been kind of bare for me. I feel that I have nothing, when I take my robe off and walk into the shower and see nothing but my feet. Scott, you don't understand my point, do you? But then again you might. I feel as if you are my older brother, but I still get upset at you for no reason. Scott, I'm sorry, I guess maybe you do understand then. I will get through this now. I will. Take care, Scott. Talk to you soon, and Robert says hi!"

"Thanks Linda," I say to myself. "It doesn't matter if you have 'A' or 'K' cup sizes. For your breast, it doesn't matter. Live life, that's all that matters." And Buzz, you might get me in trouble here, because im not sure if Linda is a blonde or not, but im going to send her a few blonde jokes.

Ok, joke time again. She is so blonde

That she was told by a doctor,since she isn't getting enough rest,

She should monitor and measure how long she slept,

So she then measured the bed, and brought a ruler to bed.

Plus, I really never got those cup stuff measurements down anyway before!

Linda sends another e-mail that I don't see until Saturday, but she reports that she starts chemotherapy on Monday. I feel like a "high" just took over me. I feel good about this, here on Friday afternoon!

My wife and children have been so supportive of me on my book and the concept behind My New Family. They continue to do what they can, by typing or talking on the phone, giving other children support.

It seems as if every day or so, we hear of cancer research testing with mice and rats. Haven't we as a country been doing this for a long time now? Call me skeptical, but does this animal really have the same genes and blood as we do? I think it's obvious over the last ten, twenty, or forty years and more, that something isn't working here with the testing of the mice for a cure. Correct me if I am wrong (and I know I will get nasty letters anyways), but I will be the first to apologize, and if it does work then let's see that data supporting this at our Mr. Senator's office to review. And if animal testing doesn't work, maybe we want to see that also. Maybe it's time to move in a different direction., in testing animals for cure for cancer, for humans. Motorola recently tested several live pigs to see if there is any risk causation of cancer while using cell phones. I would also like to see this report published at the senator's office, as I have my own doubts on the testing process and its findings. Are pigs closer to being human than any other animal out there? Do they have the same type of blood as we do the same muscles and bones? Also, while im on this topic of car phones, Can the Ceo or President of Motorola tell me face to face, and with certainly that the phones he produces do not cause brain cancer, or throat cancer, or any form of cancer? You know what, I will be waiting for that phone call, or letter from you Mr Motorola C.E.O wanting to meet me, and tell me and My New Family the truth.

A little fish like Mr. Boss in Florida found out what it is like to go up against my family. I suspect that there are a few scientists out there who are just waiting for me and my family to contact them and start questioning them, and become demanding and see the data reports. Don't get me wrong out there, I am not supporting a group of anti-government groups or anything like that, or trying to replace the system, but rather I want to keep an eye on you, and let us help and find a cure for cancer with you.

The sooner that you try and get back to your daily routines (or similar) the better it will make you feel. Don't rush or overdo it, but pace yourself and make small gains along the way. Maybe that dog needs yelling at again, something it hasn't got from you in a while, or maybe the dog needs a walk. Take it for a walk.

Listen very closely to your doctors. They are the professionals who will help in part make your recovery process as easy as possible based on your circumstances. You might be a little scared about your upcoming treatments, and that's normal. You might have questions on what to wear, whether you should eat first, or take your medications with or without the treatments. These are all good questions that you might need answers to. Ask the doctors as much as you need to. Consult with your new family for further guidance on just about anything. Your new family is out there waiting for you.

Does it mean that you will be cured? I don't know, but I sure pray it does. Does it mean it will help you mentally? Oh, I hope so much. Sometimes we may take a step back in our recovery process, but does it mean we have failed? Surely not. Just ask your sister. I would never like to be on top of that mountain of life, having everyone watch you, and you thinking that you are on top of everything and everyone. I would like to be the climber, though. I'd like to climb that mountain slowly, taking up the challenge and sometimes losing my footing and sliding down a bit, but I look up and know that I can keep going up. If you were up on top already, where can you look then, down? That's not us!

Our Job

Now that we have touched base on how I like my Fridays, I guess that I should tell you about our jobs then.

You may call it strange, but all my family members really work for the same thing: yes, fighting cancer. Our struggle to survive. This job is not like others; there is no overtime paid if you work extra hours, most days you can't call in sick, and you don't have many benefits like 401K or IRA packages. Sometimes in this job you might have to work a hundred hours a week. There are always doctor visits, and more doctor visits, chemotherapy treatments, and a variety of prescriptions to get filled.

Most times you don't have to worry about showing up at this job wearing long hair, for chemo usually takes care of that hair cut for you. Then it's back to the doctors to clean or fix a port that became clogged or dirty. Then on top of all these requirements, you must find time to eat, which means cooking, and finding the time to cook. There are times when you don't even have the taste to eat a cracker, but you still must make something to eat to help bring up your blood levels, which dropped because of the chemotherapy treatments. And of course if you have children, that is another requirement that must get met. You can't let that slide. That is just as important as all the other requirements, as is trying not to show the children how you truly feel and staying strong in front of them.

Did I forget to talk about housecleaning and food shopping? This is all part of our daily lives. The only reward is how you might feel mentally and physically. If you feel good after all this, then it's like taking home the jackpot.

So, I ask this question. How many of you reading this book right now who don't have cancer can meet these job demands? I thought so. The only ones who that come even close are the caregivers who take care of us: the wife, husband, mother, brothers, and sisters. Just try this for one week. Try cooking or helping someone go to the doctor's for a week. You will be very tired at the end, but you will feel good about your duties.

OK, it's Friday now; you are ready to just run out to that fish fry again and have a few cold ones, or could you spend just a bit of time dropping off a dinner for someone or sending an e-mail. A basket of lasagna and rolls goes along way with us. The images remain with us mentally for years. We remember that brother or sister who spent a few minutes dropping something off to someone and their children, a bag of cookies, fruit, whatever it might be.

One never knows when they might have to change jobs themselves.

You know what amazes me? Despite all the long hours that we put in fighting cancer, for the most part we will always find time to chat and talk to other family members. We find time when others say they have no time. There is always time left in a day; you just have to use it wisely.

I find it comforting when I can tell that my brothers or sisters are upset or crying, just by how they type to me. I can usually ask them to just wipe that tear off, and continue typing to me. Don't let the fear back; keep that hope going. If I can tell that the family member is upset about something, then I know they feel confident with me, and they can feel better by letting go, and lean on my shoulder with no problem. When we lose one of our family members, that screen will be just blank, and the new member who joins us knows they must have awfully big shoes to fill. Even though they might have left the job they had shared together with us, we ask that they still stay with us, watch over us, and give us strength for faith, power, and the will to continue. We are still a family; it's just that you are away from us now. Although you have been called away, we are still a family.

Growing up, did you ever wonder if you would at some point in your life get cancer? I had thought about it briefly, but felt that in my condition it wouldn't be possible. I had said that if anything, maybe when I'm seventy or eighty80 it might be a slim chance. I was well short of that, like by forty or fifty years. If I was going to get cancer, I guess now would be the best time, while I'm younger and able to fight back very aggressively. I felt like I was just entering the prime time of life. I was weightlifting a lot, running some twenty-five or more miles a week, and just beginning to live life with my family.

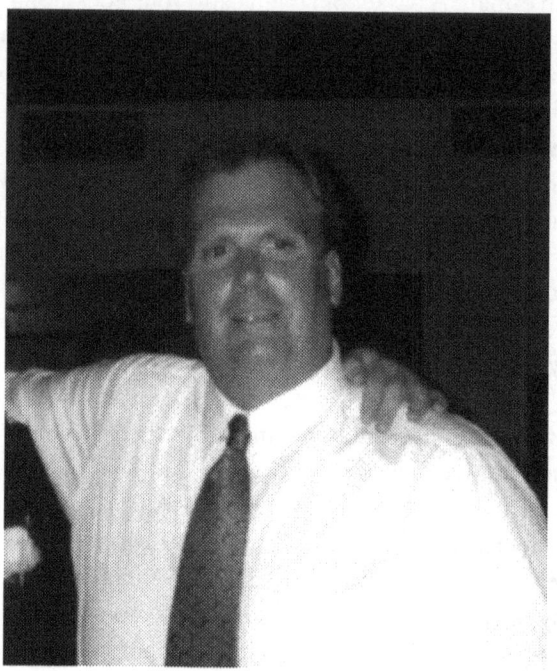

Hello, George

More than a year ago, I had a conversation with an older man who appeared to be in his late seventies or early eighties. He had cancer. He was as sharp as a pencil, I thought. When he walked, he always leaned forward, like as if he was bent over looking for something that had fallen. He looked as if he would just fall flat on his face, but he never did. While I talked with him, he would pull out a small cigar and fire it up using an old metal lighter which sent the smell of lighter fluid into the air. He always coughed a lot while he smoked, which I might add, that The scent from it almost made me cough and caused my eyes to water.

I met this old man outside in the parking lot of a small, very old grocery store, a mom-and-pop-type store, in the far northeast portion of McHenry County Illinois. It was the only store around for miles in this small, unincorporated area. So there I stood in my uniform next to my squad car in the lot talking to this man. The weather outside wasn't too bad, thirty-five or so degrees. He was wearing this very long, gray colored coat that hung well past his knees. I had originally passed by him in my squad car as he stood outside this same store, body bent over, trying to light his cigar. I turned around, pulled into the parking lot, exited the squad car, and began to walk over to him to say hi. When he saw me, he began to walk away slowly, but he had this walk about him that made him walked to the right, then to the left, but not really moving forward though. I said hi and asked him if he was OK. He turned, and looked at me directly, then spoke, "Yes, jackass, are you OK?"

His reply took me completely by surprise, and we began to talk about things now. He told me about his past and that another police officer had stopped him, kind of like I just did, and told him that it didn't look good for a person like him to be seen outside the store hanging around, and that the kids in the neighborhood would look down on him. He told me where he lived, and I verified that he lived there and hadn't been reported missing. No, not reported missing, but I think he was reported found. Found by himself, since he knew what he wanted out of life.

We continued our talk, talking about his past. He felt confident with me, knowing that I only wanted to stop and say hi, see if he needed help, and I wasn't going to give him a hard time. He again spoke of the previous statement about that earlier police officer who had told him about children seeing him. He told me that he was once a child, and that he wouldn't have looked down on an older man just enjoying life.

Being a police officer, you are trained to be neutral, open to both sides, but on this cloudy early afternoon, it was very hard for me to be anything but this, I felt sympathetic for this old guy as he spoke of the spread of his cancer, and that one day he too would join his friends and family again, who had all passed away and left him alone. I told him we should find a better spot to talk, a location that wouldn't make him feel guilty sitting there talking with me. He had thought that nobody wanted to really deal with a old man, a smelly long jacket, and a face that was not shaved, but was not dirty either. I think it actually made him look good, and tough.

Remember, this all occurred more then a year before I found out about my illness, while I was still working.

I moved my papers and items in the squad car, turned up the heat, and drove him home. To my surprise, we only had to travel across the street and four houses down. As I pulled into driveway, I parked behind an old blue Chevy four door. The car was very clean, and I noticed that there were a few newspapers on the front seat, along with two cans of corn and a can opener. He told me that he wiped off his car every other day, and that it had only 42,000 miles on it.

"I am the neighborhood," he proclaimed. "I have lived here for forty years. All the children know me here."

No police calls were coming over my radio, so I thought I would continue to and chat for a few more minutes and set a good example for law enforcement, since he already had one negative encounter in the past. He took me downstairs into his basement and showed me small toys made from wood. There were cars and trucks, houses, and small skyscrapers. He told me that the children would love to come over for one hour, sometimes with their fathers or mothers. And He told me, "I would teach them how to take a few pieces of old wood, use a few nails, and actually make that wood come to life in form of cars, trucks, etc."

He sure was creative. As I looked around at all the things he had made, I noticed the children even had painted most of them, showing a lot of care in their work. As we walked back upstairs, he told me that before he was forty years old he had never lived life. He would commute to Lake County for work, a travel time of three hours each day, there and back, and then work his normal ten-hour shift. Each day back then.

"Is this what you would call living, Scott?" he asked me. "No, never home, always working, and now my children all live out of state, all for what? He tells me. My children will visit me on Thanksgiving and Christmas. My neighbor's children visit me often; they love to build with their little hands."

He began to wipe his eyes, as they were tearing up now. I must admit I felt about the same right now.

"You know what Mr. Milkin, Milgran," he said as he tried to read my name tag on my uniform. "Oh, I'm sorry, Milliman? Then its Officer Scott Milliman?" he asked.

I tell him that we were just fine before on a first-name basis.

"I'm Scott, Scott Milliman," I told him as I shook his hand.

"I am living life now," he replied, but then we were interrupted with emergency radio traffic on my portable police radio. The dispatcher advised me that a married couple was fighting, actually fist fighting. I told this old man that I had to go now, but I would return some time and say hi. We shook hands again, and I went running out to my squad car.

As I drove to the emergency call, lights and siren on, I couldn't help but think about the call that I'm going on now and how it related to this old man that I just had met. What in life could be more important that just living it? Was this couple that I'm en route to drinking, fighting over work, fighting over money issues, fighting over love affairs? I didn't know yet, but would soon find out. You could probably bet that they weren't fighting over cancer, though. When I got there, I didn't see a clean old car sitting in the driveway, but I do see a black Lexus here.

Recently as I sat in a church services during prayer request, the pastor read a prayer from a person who asked that we pray for a good friend of his who had breast cancer. It was growing through different stages now he speaks, yet she refused to seek medical treatment. My ears popped open. I wanted to locate her and see if I could help her, guide her to support or treatment options. Not just let it take her over and keep growing, allowing it to take her on a path to destruction.

Again, I know this particular form of cancer is very personal to my sisters, but we have to try something. I will continue to pray for her, and I am going to try and locate information on her, maybe make that phone call to her. The last thing that I want to do is force something upon someone who simply doesn't want it, but I do want to make that person aware of all the options out there. It's not really my choice to intervene. Cancer has made the choice, and we can be stronger then it. Grab cancer by its ears, head butt it, and, even if it knocks you back or off your balance, get right back up there, grab its ears again, and head butt it again. Keep this up until the cancer falls back and you control its destiny.

I never really enjoyed fighting too much before. Sure, being on the police force, you were put into situations sometimes that required use of force options. I had to make decisions within a split second of time., but you had to react, I had three children and a wife at home waiting for me to pull into that driveway at the end of my shift, so I had to win those fights. and there is no difference now fighting cancer. We have to win that same fight that has been laid upon us. We must win. I remember what that old police sergeant would say at the end of the roll call, and before you hit the streets for your shift, "Hey, be safe out there."

Peaceful Feeling

During the past eight weeks, I have met with my pastors at Prince of Peace Lutheran Church, in Crystal Lake, Illinois. What started as an adult Bible-study class turned into something much different. It's now the season of fall, and usually the classes in spring and summer have higher attendance, but it's OK. Being there alone with my pastors, re-reading and learning about the Bible meant a lot to me. But we would always put aside time to discuss how my treatments for cancer were going. My pastors really wanted me to open up to them and get things off my chest and discuss them. At first we said our night prayer and included words about sin. I think at first the pastor had thought I wanted to talk about something very sinful. I explained to the pastor that over the past five years, I have been involved in political work, being a precinct committeeman in my neighborhood. I told him that I had worked hard, getting almost anyone I needed to elect into their office, going door-to-door, making phone calls, putting up signs, and so forth. I told the pastor that I had wasted so much valuable time doing this type of work and felt that my volunteer work was useless. Now I wanted to help others in a different style of life.

I asked the pastor how many sick beds he had visited or funerals he had attended for people with cancer?

He replied, "It seems that most of my visits are cancer related it seems, Scott."

I looked around in this large meeting room that we sat in with tables and chair's all organized set up, but what caught my eye were these beautiful wooden book shelves covering one whole wall, with hardly anything on them.

"Pastor," I asked, "there are a lot of support-service meetings and such here—those for marriage problems, financial problems, the children's choir, car accident victims—but is there a support group here for My New Family members who have cancer? The type of support class that meets each week—or every other week like the other groups do?"

The pastor looked at me, picked up a pen, rubbed his hands, not speaking for about twenty seconds.

He then spoke and said, "Every fall we look to others for ideas to assist our members of the church. No, Scott, we don't have anything like this, nor any of our other churches that I have belonged to in the past. I can't believe that the church has not recognized this before, Scott."

Pastor Rubeck and Pastor Schuth agreed that one hour a week would be the great, and that we could use those open book shelves to hold the latest information on cancer and information on other support groups and offers.

What better place to feel confident to meet with others than a nice big room with bookshelves and a nice warm feeling inside your church?

I don't limit this support to any certain type of religion or if you have no religious beliefs. Just find a free room to meet in and talk with other brothers and sisters once a week. Can't you smell a nice big pot of coffee brewing now and the smell of donuts in the air? (OK, must be that cop thing I am use to with donuts then, sorry.). But we can have coffee cakes, etc during our meetings.

I feel that, at least once a month during our support group meetings, a cancer specialist in cancer should attend for question-and-answer night and discuss various issues with us. It is one hour a week of feeling good, of sitting in a room not being afraid that someone might look differently at us because either we are going through chemotherapy or other treatments. No, we are having a family meeting, that's all. A meeting with My New Family members, and we won't restrict it to people who have cancer, but also caregivers, friends, and family.

Prince of Peace Lutheran Church, Crystal Lake, will be the first location for me to start. Every county should have at least one location. Even Mr. Senator's office is still an option that we are looking into as well.

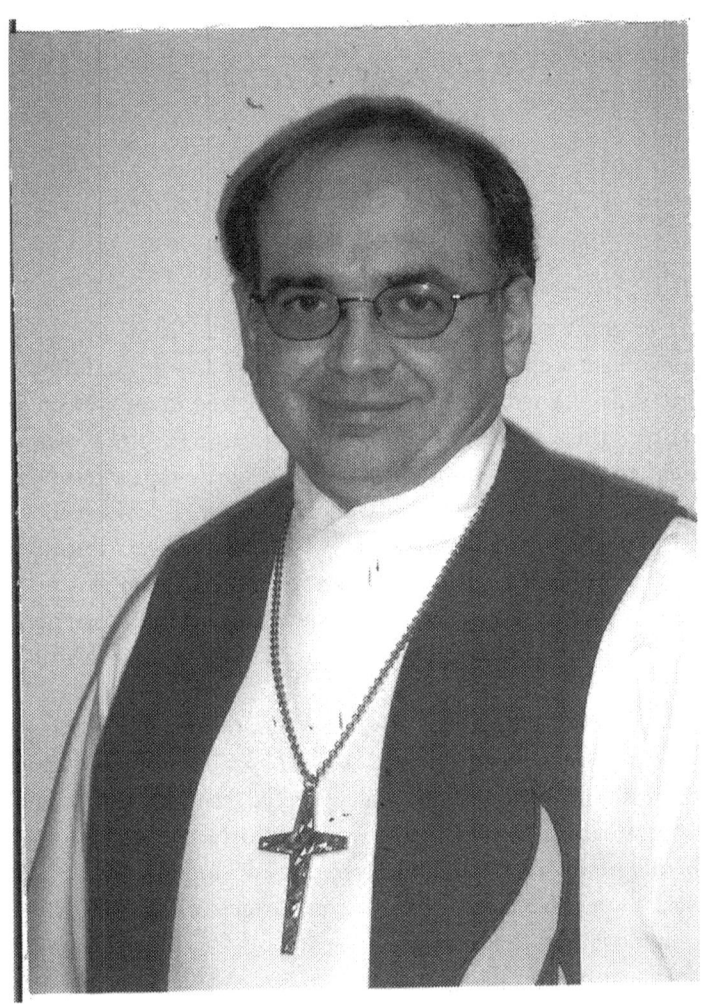

Thanks, George

I still felt so good after my discussion with that old man., smoking his old cigar. I never did get a chance to know his first name, or if he did give it to me, I can't remember. In my work, each Deputy is assigned to an area or zone for two weeks at a time, then moves to the next zone, and so on. It was almost two months since I had last seen him when I left his house that afternoon to go on a foolish family fight call. My first day back in his zone, I decided to stop in again and say hi. I'm not sure if I had questions I needed answers to inside me about this man, or just the good feeling that I had from him. I stopped and picked up a small box of cigars for him. I know, im now helping a elderly man get lung cancer by buying him a box of cigars, right? So, go ahead and write me those nasty letters too.

This time as I pulled into the driveway, I noticed a red color sports car. It looked really sharp, very expensive. As I walked past it, I didn't observe any newspapers or cans of corn on the front seat. I smiled, and felt that this old guy had really lost it now, and was probably trying to re-live his life of some forty years before with this new red sports car. After ringing the door bell, I was met by a lady who was about thirty years old and very attractive. She was scared by seeing my presence and wanted to know what was wrong. I told her nothing was wrong; I just wanted to stop and talk with the older man whom I met some eight weeks before, or so.

She replied, "Oh, you mean George?"

I said that I didn't recall his name, but he loved to smoke cigars.

"Yes, that's good old George," she replied.

She allowed me into the living room, and showed me a picture of George.

"Yes," I told her, "that's the guy."

She asked how I knew him, and I told her briefly. She stated that she was George's daughter-in-law. She said, "That old fool was hunched over trying to light a cigar on one of the busiest roads in the next county, stepped off the curb while trying to light it, and was struck and killed by a car."

My stomach sank. I have seen several fatal accidents and other death situations where people have died by being a police officer, but I never had the feeling as I had now for this old guy. I told her about my encounter with George. She told me that she and her husband, George's son, had been trying to clean his house and discovered stacks of bills and statements from doctors going back more than fifteen years. It wasn't till reading these that she had discovered George had been fighting cancer all those years, never telling his few relatives that he had cancer. She told me that George was always good at keeping things to himself and didn't like talking about personal things or to anyone about much, but he sure loved kids she said. She said George would go once, maybe sometimes twice a year, to Arizona and visit relatives.

"He never gave us any indication that he was so sick, just smoking those stupid, smelly cigars," she said.

I told her that I was sorry for their loss of George. She said at his funeral, it was very small, just a few surviving relatives and some friends. But what was odd she stated, "There were kids I never knew before there, and they all brought a toy made out of wood and placed it in his casket as they said there good-byes to George."

I asked her if she knew the meaning behind the wooden toys. She replied that one of the boys told her that George had showed him how to make something with his hands. She said that she didn't understand how he could do all this stuff, knowing he was dying of cancer, and all the doctor stuff. She happened to show me his cut out obituary from the newspaper. It said that George had died from an automobile accident. I smiled inside, handed it back to her, and thought inside me, that he didn't die from cancer; he died from the crash, a very big difference in life. I shook her hand, thanked her for her time, and began to walk out.

Upon seeing the red sports car again, I stopped, turned, and asked her, "What happened to George's blue Chevy?"

She replied, "We had it shipped back to our home in Arizona. We can sell it there after we clean the junk out of the car."

I then recalled the newspapers and cans of corn and asked her if she knew what that was about. She replied she didn't.

I pulled out of her driveway and began to leave. I was met by the next-door neighbor, who asked if everything was OK with the house. I told him briefly yes, and he stated that the neighborhood would miss George. They would no longer see him sitting in his old car, down the cul-de-sac by the lake, wiping off his car with towels, always, or reading the newspaper. He would actually take a can of vegetables, open it up, and eat directly from the can, throwing a few nibbles out for the birds to eat as well.

"He was one good old guy, that George was," the neighbor told me.

"Yes, he was," I replied.

I still have that box of cigars in the squad car with me. From time to time, I would take a good whiff of the box, and it brings me back to seeing and hearing that old man.

The cigar box is wood, you see, George, and you somehow built this too.

Another Friday has come upon us already. This particular Friday is not a usual winter day. It's nice and sunny and seventy degrees. I will have to take advantage of this unusual winter day. It's been almost four weeks now since I last heard from Jennifer, a sister who has been suffering from cancer. We usually chat via e-mail for a while. However, today I get a reply from her husband, who reported that her cancer has taken on a new growth, and that she had emergency surgery on or about October 19. He reports that she is still in ICU at the hospital and has had several more seizures.

Our brother Buddy is now recovering from yet another surgery at Duke University, where the doctors had found new growth again in the tumor. I talk with Buddy daily on the phone and update Buddy's wife, Kim, on the news about Jennifer, as Kim and Jennifer also e-mail each other. All my other contacts are all reporting progress this week, and I tell them to have a great weekend.

I'm going to try and get outside today and suck up as much warm air as I can. This week I am on chemotherapy, and I have my own ups and downs. I'm somewhat tired, and I have an upset stomach at times. But none of this can interfere with my dream, My New Family. I locate information on the lady from our church who had breast cancer and is refusing to do anything about it, that I had spoken of before. I forward on to her the names of a few sisters and their phone numbers, in case she would like to discuss treatment options with them. I just don't want to see her go through this without doing anything. She should at least just simply talk to another sister for support help. I have no fish fry to go to tonight, and I'm not a clubber type person, so I will end this Friday inside my home with my family, take my chemotherapy after my e-mailing is complete, and pray for all of us.

Throughout our life, I'm sure that we have all felt a level of accomplishment when we did something. It could be from getting good school grades, to securing a job, a family, or so forth. These are all great, but the smallest of a daily activity can be felt as a huge accomplishment too. For those who can get enough strength to get off the couch or chair or pull themselves to another side of the couch or to a different chair, this is also a huge accomplishment. That would feel good doesn't it? It's the same feeling as the person who got good grades or the one who secured that job so he can support his family. Let me know how you changed something in your life to meet that accomplishment. If you are having difficulty reading, let someone read you this book. As you lie back and relax, let your ears open up to hearing that email sound that alerts you that a new message has come in from a brother or sister or a phone call. These are all major accomplishments.

I was always proud of the letters of commendation that I received over the past years from the sheriff's office. I have always been known as someone who doesn't hide his feelings, so here I go. I say bullshit to all those letters. Yeah, they were for line of duty accomplishments. Sure, it helped at the time and made me feel good that my work had paid off. But nothing at all can come close to the sense of feeling accomplishment as I have now, the fighting against cancer and my writing of this book. Hearing hundreds—thousands—of your daily fighting-cancer stories is so much more rewarding. Having the willpower to stay in the den, day after day, e-mailing to you all so that we can be joined as a family, talking about this illness that's in our bodies, what it has done to us, and our long list of family members in the past makes it worth the fight.

Guy's, do you know how much pain I'm actually in, as I sat with you all this morning, for the lunch special in the garage for the Sheriffs office? I know that probably when I go home, im going to pay the price for eating like this while I'm on chemo today. I wore this hat today because I can't control my eyes watering when I see you all. I saw each one of my ladies from records look at me, and I tried so hard to stand straight, walk in pace, and smile for you girls, but it hurts. Today it hurts pretty bad, but I know that if I could just show you all in person that we can fight this, it might help you or others one day. A white shirt that sat across from the table from me, made a comment to me this morning that he wished I would come back to work at the Sheriffs dept, and since I wont be, that's ok because things happen. But wait, I know for a fact that I will return to the sheriffs dept. I have no doubt of that. By seeing your face and your stupid comment to me in regards to me being able to "work inside a police dept answering phones some where", reassured me on how much of a *&$%) you really are. I will return back to my job in full duty, and I can honestly say this today as I take my chemotherapy that I 'WILL BE BACK"

If you are helping a family member now, you should receive that commendation. It is here that we must re-learn about life, and what is truly important to us, what makes us feel good naturally. So go and visit your new family member now.

Wouldn't it be nice one day to have several brothers and sisters stand side by side with a scientist as he reads to the nation the cure for cancer? Then that day, a letter of commendation should be issued to them all.

Denial is not an option for us. It doesn't make our disease go away, and it doesn't help on our recovery process. It is what it is, and we must take the steps to fight the illness. It doesn't matter if you are four years old or eighty, we still have to get ourselves mentally ready for this battle and take it on. The only difference in age is the strength and endurance, but what remains the same is life. That is what matters, life, time on earth to be with others. The ladies who I work with at the records department at the sheriff's office have taught me so much about life that I thought I never would have known. Ladies, As I sat at that same table eating lunch today, I saw all your faces, felt your hugs, saw your smiles, and I really wanted to come here today to join you for lunch, and let you see first hand what your prayers and thoughts have done for me. I am walking proof, that you helped me through my battles each day as I woke up, and maybe a bit more important, that somehow help me to reach tomorrow. Out of my five-day work week, I try to stop up at the records department three or four times a week and take a chocolate candy bar that they pass out to each person who wants one, and stop in and say hi. I never used to eat chocolate or have a taste for it until I met those girls. I would eventually take a few extra candy bars and I would then pass them out to people I met on calls during the night, as an exhibit to show them I care for them as well. It could be a small child lost, a husband and wife fighting, or simply a traffic stop. The way that the person feels after receiving this token is so positive. Thank you, ladies, for showing me this gift of life. I love you all, and will try to continue kicking this cancer out of me, so that I could return one day, and get that candy bar each day before I hit the road.

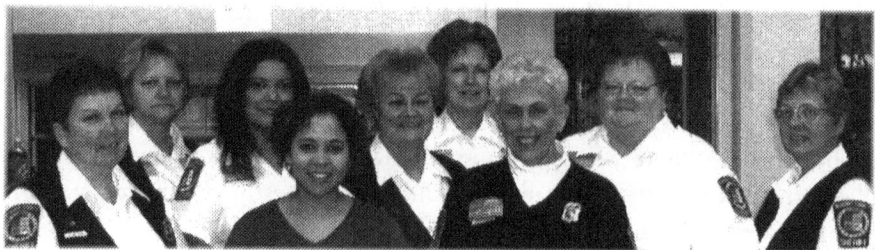

Just recently I have spoken to a friend of my family whothat I have known for some time now. He has been diagnosed with lung cancer. In talking about the upcoming treatments, he felt so confident talking to me about life. He was, of course, very nervous, as the doctors wanted treatment to begin within the next two weeks. I told him how important it is to listen and follow the doctor's instructions. Two weeks later he called me as he began his treatments.

"As I cough, you know, Scotty, the chemotherapy makes me sick, and I feel very scared. But, man, I don't have to tell you, Scotty, about that stuff, you know it already, I guess we both are there now."

I tell him yes, we both are fighting the same thing. Then it sank into me, this is my new brother. After talking to him for almost an hour, he said he would call me after his next visit in about two weeks. I tell him that I will call him well before that date, and he should feel free to call me before as well, just to chat and say hi.

Every day that passes, I feel that My New Family is out there gaining support. Even if it's one person at a time, that's OK. One person is still a heartbeat that we can listen to.

The Bully

In writing this book and in my group discussions, I have attempted to limit myself to time on talking about a particular experience with cancer so as not to soak up the time from others. Sure, I will from time to time bring my own experience up, but it helps me with my daily fight to discuss it, even if it is just for a short moment. I know what it feels like to discuss the pain and suffering from something that has been placed into your body to attack us, cancer. What happened recently, though, really took me off guard, and it felt as if I was pushed back up against a wall by some big bully. But this time I fought back with an enormous amount of power and spoke my words, lifted myself off my back, and fought back. I've been doing this with all of you in my mind, through this whole process. Let me explain now, who that bully is, and what they were telling me to do.

There is no doubt that over the past several long months, I have gone through several emotional and physical changes in my own life. I realized at some point that I have this "open-hearted love" to help my new family, and I have worked very hard at establishing this. Yes, there were days when that it was so hard to type on my computer keyboard and to send e-mails to others who maybe were not as sick at the time as I was at the time, or may have been even sicker. But I continued my typing, asking how their day was going, how are their treatments going? Encouraging them to keep pushing, sending words of hope and will. During this week that I spoke to this bully, I had several sisters and brothers in the hospitals going through severe treatments. I asked their relatives to please read my e-mails to them, and let them know I'm still here and typing to them, and will be when they get out of the hospital. Several different states may separate us, but love and commitment don't create a distance between us. We were together. I have lost one brother and one sister this week, and I felt their loss, and now I won't receive an e-mail from them this week. I still believe that because they were called away; they didn't go away. I'm sure that you all are still with me—and us—and will always be there, helping us to defeat the enemy: cancer.

This week is a bit tougher than most past weeks. The snow is finally falling now, and soon it will be the holidays again. It has been too bitterly cold out to go walking. I understand by my new approach on life that it would be a roller-coaster at times, having sisters and brothers doing well one week, while others might have taken a turn for the worse. I understand this and am fully prepared for all this. This will not stop me from writing my book, and it especially will not deter me from my daily contacts with all My New Family members. No, it won't stop or change me. Even when that stupid bully continues to try and change my ways of thinking, it will not affect me here.

Well, the bully couldn't face me, face-to-face, but rather used the telephone as the weapon of choice against me. I had my own medical treatments this week and handled them very well. Sure, it gets to you a bit, but what the heck, it was OK. So, the bully wanted to know how this past week went for me. I was a bit surprised that I even got this phone call from this bully, since this bully was not a contributing factor in my day to day recovery process, and even less with helping out my own family, here at home..

After a very short discussion, the bully went for my throat right away, saying, "You know what, Scott, I think you should stop speaking with all those sick people on the computer. Doesn't it make you mentally sick listening to their problems as well?"

I replied that I don't care how sick I might be or the condition of any My New Family members, I will continue to speak my thoughts and feelings every day and encourage others to do the same. How can this bully ask me to shut a door on another family member like this? No, it will not happen, and all it did was piss me off more and allowed me to sit and type more today to my family members. Yep, this person doesn't have a clue about life if she hasn't talked to my brothers and sisters in this world. Yes, I think one day I might be speaking to her on the computer, as maybe a new sister, and I will not shut the door on her, as she did to me and My New Family. But I will ask that she open the window of life first, begin to help those like my family members, and then one day open her door.

How Can I Show You This?

This holiday season is one that I have been waiting for since my surgery with brain cancer. I know that I have touched base on the bully story in my life, but it doesn't stop there.

No, I have tested my thoughts about this bully with several other persons who that I call friends. I decided to call a female friend who that I and my family have known for some twenty years. After calling my friend, she asked me about my progress and how the treatments for the past several months had been going for me. I simply replied by saying, "Oh, you mean the cancer treatments?"

She tells me yes and that I must be doing very well, since after surgery she really never heard from us.

I paused for a moment, smiled to the phone headset, and thought to myself, *I'm right on target.* I know exactly what just happened, but give her time to reply back to me.

She stated, "I know that you must have a lot of your police officer friends stopping by all the time and taking care of you, but we need to get together for dinner, all of us."

I don't want to say anything bad about my friends, especially those who I have spent my lifetime basically with, but this just proves to me one of the reasons that I sit and write this book. I want others to realize what a family is about and how to take care of others in need—offering the simplest things in life, sharing a book, car ride, or a phone call. Yes, there were a lot of fellow police officers who had stopped by to see me and the wonderful ladies in records who never forget a holiday greeting card to me.

Ladies, I still read the words you all took the time to write to me.

Yes, my friend, you were right. There was the Mattison family and their wonderful baskets of fresh vegetables and that music disc that you gave me. Did you know, Tim that I would listen to the music on the days when I was feeling so worn out from the chemotherapy and that I needed a nap? I couldn't get past the third song before I would sleep peacefully and could almost feel the chemo working away at where it needed to, killing the cancer growth. Thanks for being a brother, Tim.

Brother Mike Lucas, I remember your visits and taking me out to see what is being built in our city and or those rides to get me out of the house to breathe some fresh outdoor air. Mike, your magazines that you would also bring over helped me to concentrate on reading again and the updates on job changes which helped me get back in the groove quicker to try and help me return back to the "World of Law Enforcement".

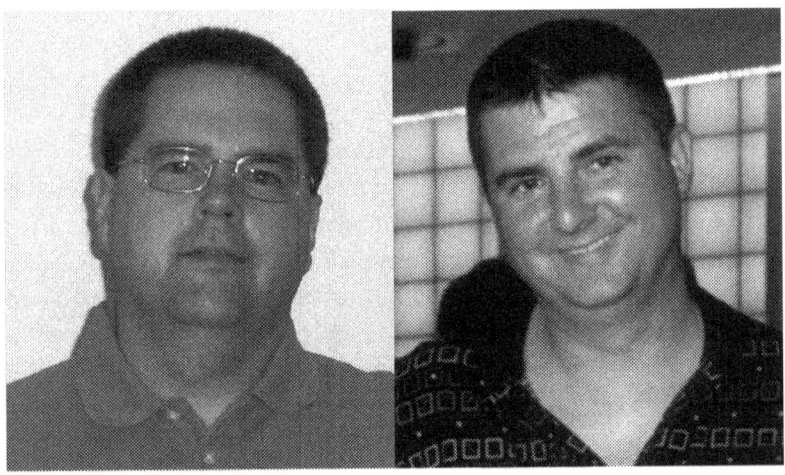

Brother Bodden, taking me out to the movies felt like a million bucks, and maybe the girls you showed me at Hooters before dinner helped as well! I loved seeing the movie 'Eight Mile". Everyone in the theater thought we were crazy, being almost 40 years old, and see the movie. His words in some of his songs are very true. And in either case, we had a great time watching the movie, wolfing down a bucket of popcorn with you, and forgetting about what I must have to go back home and do. Take my chemo. I also realized that this time together, would mean a re-charge for Wendy. Maybe she could sit back and just relax tonight, and not have to worry about watching over me for one night. Thanks buddy.

Brother Dave Nash, thanks for not allowing me to say no, when you would stop by on a Saturday and pick me up for lunch. This is after you would already work some 60 hours at Motorola. The inspiring words that you spoke of on the child mentor program is great. Keep up the good job. That little boy that you take out really looks up to you I bet. Im sure that he looks toward seeing you that one day a week, just as I am to see Pastor Rubeck and Pastor Schuth Thursday night for one hour.

There were all my great neighbors who took turns cooking for my family for a few weeks while I was very ill, my supervisors who would call and take me out to lunch, and friends who I haven't talked to in years, stopping by picking me up for lunch as well.

The phone calls, the visits, the lunch, greeting cards, these are all examples of how you were brothers and sisters to me. Tom and Anita, Gary and Heidi, Dan and Ann, Jim and Kelly, Jon and Jan, Jill and Matt, Mike and Darla, these are just a few brothers and sisters who made my recovery possible. I do have a question for you guys, though. Who took my twelve-pack of Miller Lite from me? I will need that back one day soon!

And my own family supporting me, finding the medical treatment that I need, always being there for me, and showing me what it is like to have a brother and sister. Now I can share you with the world, your inspirations that you allowed me to open and share with others. As my professor told me in the police academy, "If you could change one life, if you could take one person from a negative situation into a positive one, you would just have completed a full year's of hard work." I think you are all ready to work many, many, years. I have just a few more pages to write, and then I will let you go and start your new membership into My New Family.

Can You Tell I'm Back to Typing Again?

As I sit trying to eat my breakfast, which in itself is a hard task for me today, I begin to read the local newspaper. I usually don't read the paper anymore. Since I live in the northwest suburbs of Chicago, the paper is filled with deaths and other bad news.

Today there is a picture and a large article of our local senator. The article reads that the state senator is recovering from walking pneumonia. The article reports that he has had pneumonia four times before, and that the doctor wanted to hospitalize him, even though he was up and walking around. He feels good, the article states.

Upon reading the article, I looked in the obituaries section and located several persons who have passed away from cancer. Ages were reported from eighteen to seventy-three years old. Several were listed with no picture at all.

A few days later you, Mr. Senator, returned back to work. I was happy to hear that. I was also glad you fully recovered from your pneumonia. You could see for yourself how difficult it was when you were ill, but look at the public awareness that you received. You were in the newspaper, and thousands of people read the article. I must tell you that I have already spoken about you and the other senators before, several chapters ago in my book. It was on how you, Mr. Senator, could be such a huge assistance, bringing attention and up-to-date information on cancer for My New Family. All the public awareness programs, the grants, the marathons, the cookie sales—all these things could help raise money for cancer awareness, and also the money donated from directly out of our own pockets (pockets that have several holes in them, very worn out, but still trying to donate what we can to help with cancer detection, awareness, and research). I know that I have spoken on how you, Mr. Senator, will play a part in the program to fight cancer, or at least supply us a place that we can go to, read it ourselves, and try to be relaxed.

I hope that you get My New Family's ideas about our fight for the cure and more intervention from the federal and state government. I am not taking advantage of, or making light of, the pneumonia that you had recently, but rather making you more aware of our needs. I realize that the article a few weeks ago reported that on Monday you had to cancel a few meetings because you were recovering from pneumonia, but do you have any idea how many meetings or appointments we must keep that we can't cancel during our battle with cancer?

In the world today, there are various countries that for various reasons to reason are at war among themselves. Our country is fighting in Iraq, this would be the second such war in about ten years. Upon watching the news reports and newspaper articles on the upcoming war, there appears to be a big difference of public opinion as to whether or not we should be in Iraq at this point. The one thing that stands out on the news reports is the common public discussions on the loss of American soldiers.

Our president spoke today, and stated, "The loss of one soldier is one soldier too many."

I didn't have to be a past or current member of the armed forces to understand this phrase because it is true; these men and women are fighting hard for our country and our rights.

I totally respect our government and our country, including all branches of the armed forces. What I want to show is how much our country will spend in dollars for protecting our country and its citizens. We have heard from my past writings in this book, on about how many men and women come down each year with cancer, and the numbers of us who have lost our lives in this battle. If we paid as much attention and money to the war against cancer as the war against terrorism, wouldn't we have a cure? To the cause, and the cure for this war causing agent, cancer, I still can't figure out mentally, and now physically why we don't have this answer? And how many wars have been fought since the first cancer case was discovered? Yes, you probably asked in your mind which war, the armed forces war with countries or with cancer? Take your pick, but the number of lost brothers and sisters who fatally fell in by their bedsides, battle after battle, is just too hard, and too great of numbers for me to imagine at this point.

Some of my brothers and sisters are also members of the armed forces, and they sometimes must have to fight two different wars: one to protect our country and the other to protect their body from cancer. If our country needs to build the latest equipment designed by our top engineers and scientists, like Stealth Bombers, global tracking, and unmanned tanks, why the heck can't we discover the cure for cancer?

With permission, I now will enclose just a small percentage of the e-mails that I have received since My New Family started. As you read them, please excuse any spelling or grammar errors. Please prepare your Gloria Jean cup of tea, coffee, or other drink, and find an area where you can just sit back, sip, and relax while you read the e-mails, and get a hint of what we might do to help each other.

By setting our sights on something, most of the time we can accomplish it. I was told this time and time again, whether it was in school by a teacher, or growing up by my mother. I didn't spend much time thinking about this, though, and if things did happen, I would think it was just part of life. Sometimes you win; sometimes you lose.

I do set my sights now on this. My goal is to beat cancer and live a long life with my family and friends. Of course, beating cancer doesn't ensure you a long life table. You can walk out the door one day and be involved in a car crash or become ill with some other illness. So by saying this, I can't leave each morning worrying I might get killed in a car accident. If I fly for that business trip, I might not return? But waking up each morning knowing that I have cancer and what I can do about it, I can increase my life expectancy.

If a doctor looks at me and tell me I have only twelve weeks left, every day beyond those twelve weeks would be an accomplishment for me. So I would set my goals, not by weeks, but by years. Every year I would tell myself that I need to do this or that next year and not allow anything to interrupt that. I don't set any unrealistic goals, though—just that I want to live. That's the first goal to set my sights on.

I don't want to say the following statement to upset anyone, but the good Lord must wait a long time before I go. I know from my own personal experiences that I can alter my physical and mental state during the treatments of chemotherapy and surgery. Some by choice. Exercise and eating healthy can help this out. Remember that for each year you smoke, it puts another nail in your coffin, or something like that. Well, I use the same theory. For every day that I can exercise for twenty minutes or more, I take a nail out of the coffin. It sure works for me mentally.

It felt like maybe I spoke of this somewhere earlier in this book, so sorry if I did, but it's a crucial point I feel in fighting cancer. The mind makes the body do what it wants it to do. So if we tell our minds that we are going to beat cancer and set our sights on this, I strongly believe that it helps. Sure, there are some of us who because of the advanced stage of their disease can't set too many goals. But it is here that My New Family members should step up and assist. We all are only human. Maybe by making that spinach or salad to make others feel better, you can help those people set their sights and goals. They might get a little extra perk that day, and who knows? Maybe tomorrow they might get outside for a walk, something they haven't done in a while.

Here are a few more e-mails that I wanted to share with you and some pictures of My New Family members and great friends you help others..

Enjoy.

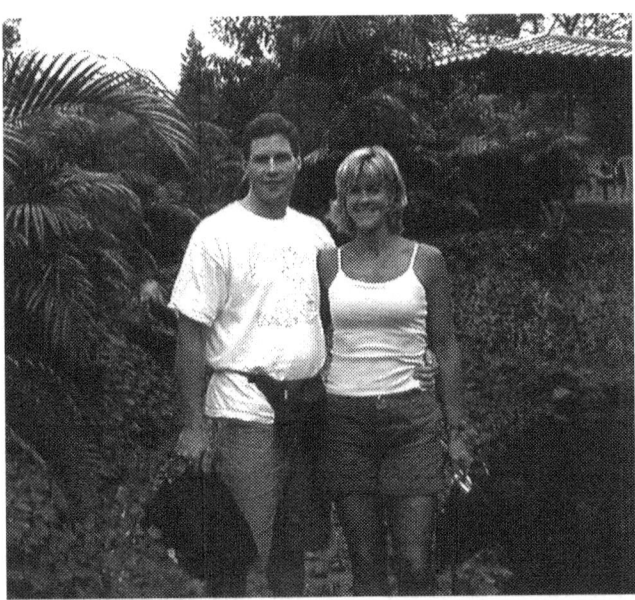

"Dear Friends, tonight I found out that a good friend of mine has got cancer throughout his body., every vital organ has cancer. He has an enlarged heart….He was recently married just in July and is only thirty-three years old. He and I grew up together side by side, he is like a brother to me and this news is just taken me by such shock."
They believe in Prayer, so I am asking all of you to take a moment today and say a prayer for Joel.
West Virginia

"Thanks for checking in. This week I feel great. And truly feel like I can get back to work. I've been wondering lately what type of Brain tumor do you have?"

Illinois

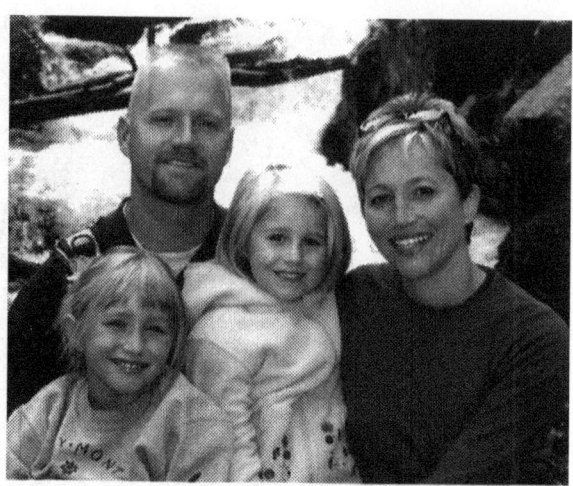

Children in Need of Rides Request.
Submitted to Amtrak for consideration, and they reply:
"Amtrak is lawfully mandated to achieve an ever-increasing percentage of cost recovery from revenues;, we are unable to honor requests for charitable contributions or free or reduced rate transportation, Regards, Amtrak."

I reply,
Give me a break;, you have got to be kidding me. You would rather allow your train to drive from Chicago to Orlando with forty-five empty extra seats, and then allow five or so sick and ill children the chance to ride the train to Disney World, a chance that might never come to these little ones. Most are unable to fly due to their illness. This is my dream, and I will make sure that I don't let it fall to the wayside for these little kids. I hope you enjoy your "Percentage of cost recovery from revenues."

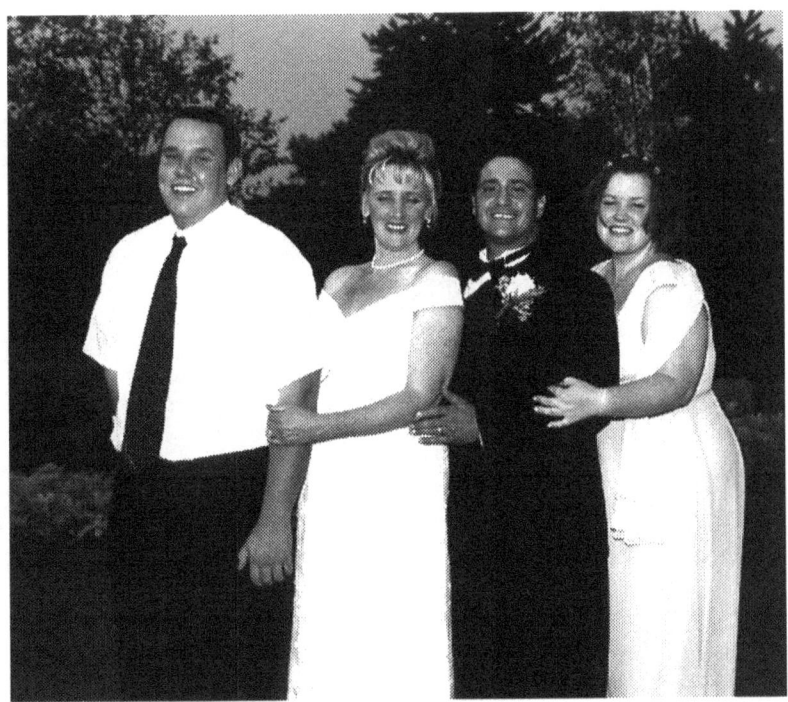

There are many signs around us. Early this morning I heard the pleasant coos of the morning doves. It will be nice to feel the warm sun, smell the fresh spring air, and see the world around us start to show signs of new green life again. Hope you are doing well and we look forward to seeing you walk in and take a candy bar from the jar and chat with us again.
Jan, Lori, Sandy, Diane, Lisa, Pat, Barb, Janet. (My friends in records)

"Great to hear from you, Scott. I'm getting back into the swing. My boss is in town for the week, so it's been a little crazy ☹."
Washington

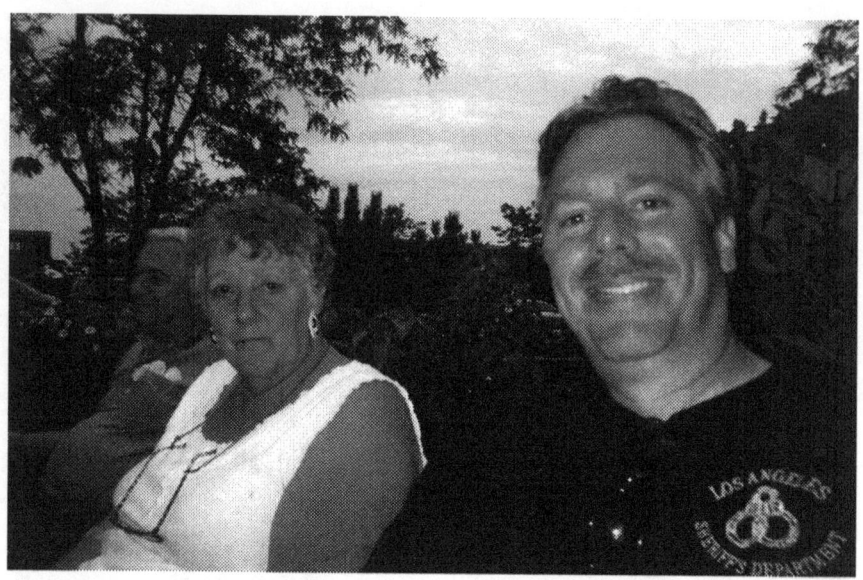

"Hey guys, just a note to say that Buddy had a good day today, The first time he's had a good day in months."
My pal, Buddy.

"Thank you both for replying back to me. I know it's been very difficult for you to continue typing probably. I thank you for still being a sister/brother for us still fighting this battle."
New Zealand.

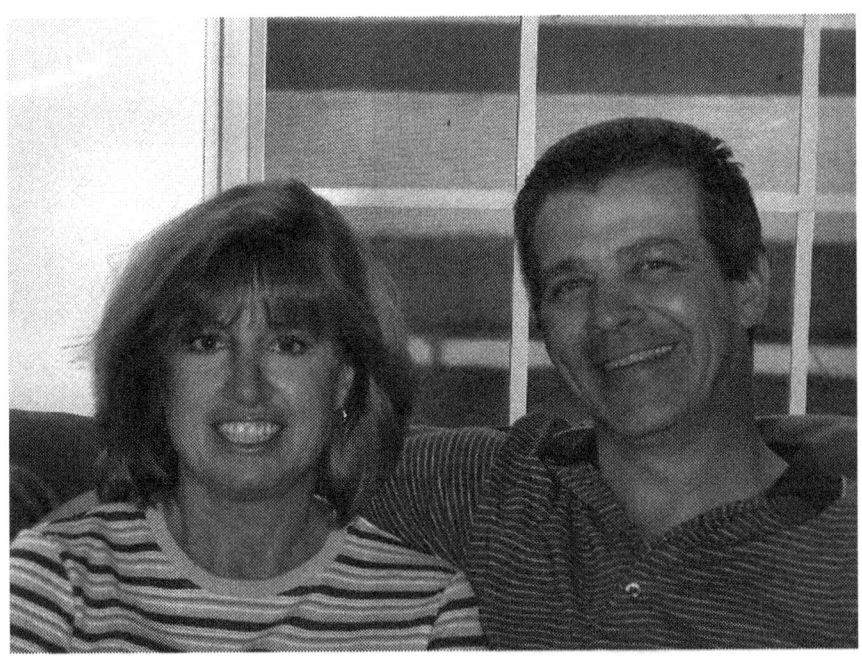

"Dear Scott, Thanks for your email. I can still remember how Deane was post-surgery. Deane is an inspiration for many people; his courage and strength is unbelievable. I am so proud of him."
"Just continue to keep positive. My best to you for a full recovery."
Ohio

Hi Scott,
"Thanks for sending us an email. We live in northern California. We are still missing Scott, but we always will. He was a fighter and we are so proud of all that he did.
Peter and I wish you the best hope that the chemo is still shrinking the tumor. We remember it well, how nervous it can be when it is time for another MRI, just hang in there, Scott, be positive and keep fighting."
Peter and Sandy (on the loss of their son Scott)

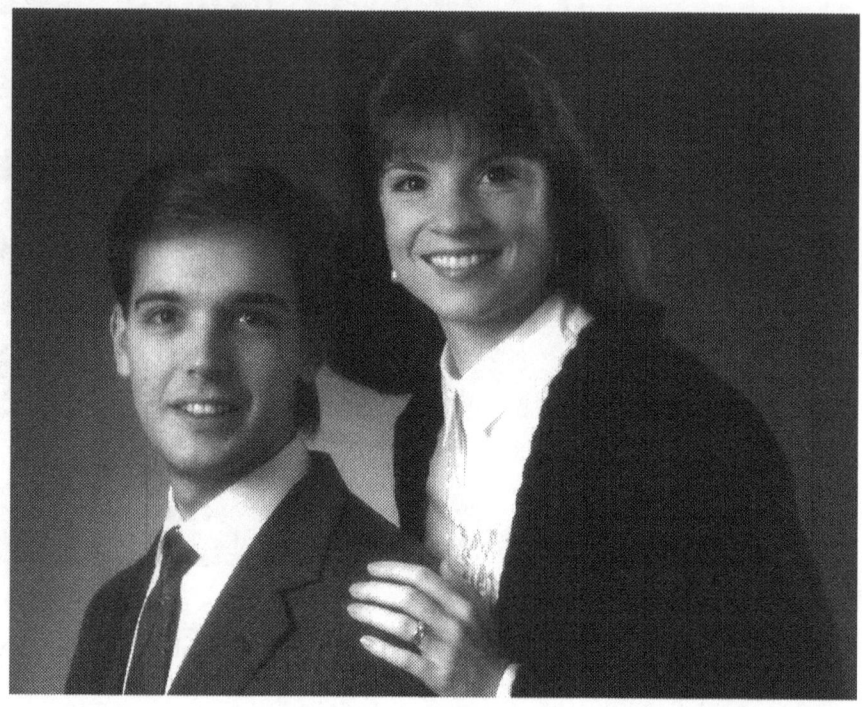

As I type this to my fellow workers at the sheriff's office.

"Good morning. I know I sent you all, those that I work with a letter probably two months ago or more. It was a thank you for all you have done, and it also was about trying to install into us the meaning of life, love, family. Remember? Taking those few extra minutes a day to give love to those whom you are so close to, or not even close at all. Your family, wife, husband, girl/boyfriends (or both), and fellow workers. If I was to take a poll on those of you who take that extra time to share a moment with your family, I think the percentage would have changed to a high, much higher level now. I can feel it as well."
OK, you're thinking, *Where in the heck is this going?*
Just a quick refresher note, if I may speak.

I read the other day from someone in Texas, in the city of Dallas, that they have a local ordinance that could be enforced if they chose. by a police officer. Let me read it to you.

"It is forbidden that anyone walking about aimlessly, with no apparent purpose, lingering around, hanging around, lagging behind, idly spending time, delaying, sauntering, and or moving slowly about, is in violation of this ordinance."

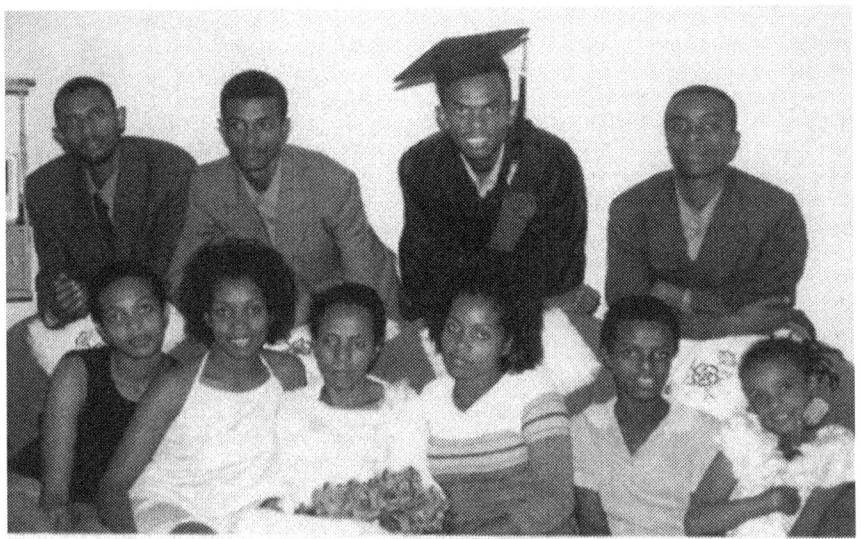

Does this ordinance describe some of your best-spent days?
Enjoy life, love your family, forgive the past, and live tomorrow.
Love Scott Milliman.

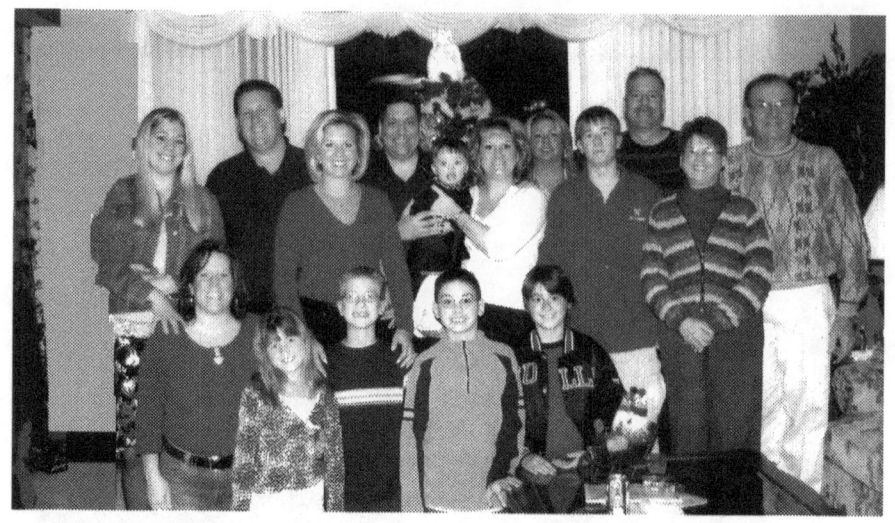

Just like a professional baseball game only goes nine innings, this book too shall have to end. You can pitch all you want for the first eight and a half innings, but if you don't have a good closing pitcher and the help from your team members, all your eight innings of pitching don't mean nothing if you lose the game. You will get a loss credit in your standings.

It is the same with this book that I spent so much hard time writing, and for all those who I proudly spoke of, and our dreams. I brought this to the eighth inning. I had a difficult time trying to close this out, and reach that win column.

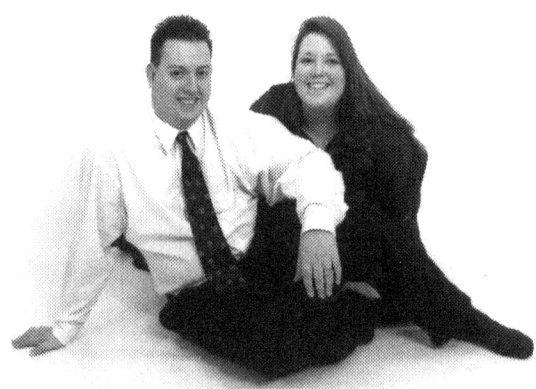

Stuart and Jennifer McIntosh, from Forever Dreems entered my life and became My New Family members. Stuart was that closure that I needed.

I am one person, but I feel that I speak for thousands of us, and we all thank you for all those nights that you were out late working on this project, and then going to work the next day feeling sleepy all day. Thank you for the nights that I took you away from Jennifer and missing your dinners together. Thank you from all of us who will sit back and read this book, Stuart.

And my long distance best friend, Bill Erfurth. Thank you, Bill, for always keeping me positive and realizing that tomorrow will always be there for me when I wake up, because I will see your e-mail when I wake up, and I can go after my dreams of writing. T.N.T. brother, T.N.T.

After reading today's e-mail, I type:

"As the New Year comes in this morning, there is a stillness on my computer, a small, soft quiet, like the period after shutting down the computer at night.

It is not how we are accustomed to it. It is a quiet that will remain. For now they have told me that Jenny has passed away.

Among those of people who move about when the day has begun, Jennifer and Jose were either home or at a hospital taking care of their business." There were many of us that had kept that special time each day to wait and check our emails, sending them back and forth. Sometimes one would smile, and others would walk away very sad after sending their e-mails. But the communication keeps on. Everyone is trying to fight the battle against cancer. At times during the day, it is a bitter war.

Some of you have no such battles to fight, but continue to join our battle and help the wounded. I thank you so much. Don't give up on us; keep us strong so we can help each other as well. I know that you have your own careers, but you've made a huge impact on all of us with your few free minutes.

Our family guarantees the rights of "minority" groups, those of certain races, backgrounds, men, and women…shit, we don't care, and we are all one of the same in this battle, the fight of our lives against in cancer.

They tell me about this new Botox stuff that they have invented to make people look younger; Viagra to help increase the sex drive; cloning; I can keep going on, but where is the cure for cancer? Since day one when I found out about my near death cancer, I have never said, "Why me?" or "Poor me." Nope, it's all about us! We are all one group. As my friends Buddy and Bill continue to kick the shit out of the cancer, it gives me more happiness to sit and type. Buddy, who has been through several surgeries and chemotherapy after chemotherapy, only to keep giving one hundred percent! (Not sure yet why he likes eating this buttermilk pie stuff, so I will have to send him some good pizza!).

Kim, Noah, Hanna, and Buddy's whole family have been waiting months at a time to come home from the hospitals, just to see his balding, smiling face—love ya bud.

In conclusion, I just wanted to bring this past year into a more positive year. While closing the previous year, we will never forget our brothers and sisters who have passed.

I am not a theologian, and I do not understand those things that many men talk about, and write about of the hereafter. I'm not quite sure how things will be when my own time comes to join Jose, Jennifer, John, Dad, Phil, and others who have passed before me. I do not have any definite information whether I will be permitted to have a computer with e-mail up there to be able and communicate with My New Family members. Even though we haven't seen each other before, I'm sure their faces will seem familiar. I do believe that I will receive a lot of e-mails up there also and will enjoy that time as well."

In closing today, may each day bring better health results for you, both mentally and physically! May each one of us find comfort within each other. It takes seconds to help bring peace and comfort into another's life, yet it took many months of pain and fighting to prove this.

Scott Milliman

Well, after leaving several phone calls and messages with Mr. Senator's office, I was finally told that his office is too busy to handle something like what we want to do," but thanks anyways."

My book was supposed to be finished by now, and I still had left this ending chapter open to finish my quest. Prince of Peace Lutheran Church did give me the go ahead and will dedicate a large room for us each week to get the program off the ground and running. The pastors were not that concerned about religious backgrounds and beliefs, but wanted you to come in a relaxed environment and learn more about life by becoming a new brother or sister. then anything else can teach you.

I am closing my book now. It's extremely hard and difficult to think of this thou. It seems as if I have so many "open chapters' in my book to be completed yet. What do I have to do, to make you realize and be heard of what needs to be done? If I have brought you this far in life, to this final chapter of my book, then you already know what you need to do. If you are still unsure, remember don't give up. Think positive. Eat well. Push a bit harder each week, reassure that you are in charge. Say hi to someone that you have never met before in words of encouragement email. Shake that hand of a stranger. Thank Rush St Lukes and Evanston Northwestern Hospitals for allowing us, My New Family, to meet Dr Byrnes and Dr Paleologos. Thank God for giving us this power to connect, Thank my own family for not giving up on me, and pushing me to that next day. Thank all my friends and workers who helped grab my arm, and pulled me up.

I still have a few missing members, that I miss talking to. Bill, way up in Northern Wisconsin for example. Where you been? And, how are you?

How about one more blonde joke for you all?

Ok, She is so blonde that when she heard that 95 % of all

Crimes are committed at home, she hurried up and sold the house.

Also, one more thought for the greeting cards on a happy marriage,

"congratulations on your wedding day!
Too bad no one likes your husband.

Ok, that was bad..how about a simple friendship one then?

'We've been friends for a very long time..
What do you say we stop?

In my final closing words, I have been informed of a new brother today join-ing My New Family. He has been diagnosed with multiple myeloma cancer. This addition to the family is somewhat surprising to me. I met this new brother with arms wide open. I visited his home, which was near me. I brought a basket of fresh vegetables and tomatoes, spaghetti noodles, garlic, and a wonderful music disc to listen to. Yes, just like brother Tim had brought me before to help me. I knew who this brother was before I even arrived. We sat and talked openly in his living room on the upcoming treatments and how scared he was. He couldn't fig-ure out how he got the cancer, but more importantly he didn't understand why there isn't an easier cure and treatments for this. He showed me an article on his type of cancer dating back to the late 1970's, where it had talked about certain treatments helping this form of cancer. I believe he said this information came from one of the largest cancer hospitals in the Midwest. I shook my head and didn't understand either. We both gave each other words of encouragement and promised that we would keep in contact with one another regularly, which we did.

Mr. Senator became my new brother on that morning. Do I have to say any-thing further? Do I have to sit and write any more pages in my book? No, my writing is over; it is now time to continue with my quest and help another My New Family member, and I hope you will as well. I'm sorry, Mr. Senator, that you have cancer also now, I truly am.

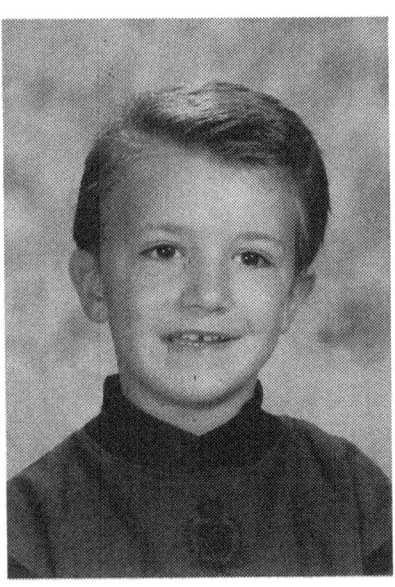

MICHAEL

I'm hours away from the final draft on my book, but must put the brakes on this, An important project of mine, in printing of My New Family book.

I knew that this so call ending of typing my book will have to end, and I did try. But I can't without telling you, Michael that this new drug out here called Temodar, which is made by Schering-Plough has been doing wonders for me, and others with brain cancer, to kill off the cancer cells it needs to. I have been so excited about this news Michael, but I would tell someone walking down the street, they might not jump up and down with glee and happiness but I know by telling you, I could feel a tear drop fall and land all the way down here on top of us.

Michael, your mom and dad are doing ok, are very proud of you, although they still miss you so much, as im sure your grandparents do, and everyone else that you had touched in your short life little guy.

You have two brothers now, but wait-I don't have to tell you that, as I'm sure you watch over them daily. Michael, your family, the Glueckert's, The Iscra's, the Rothermels, the Zekens have been such an inspiration to My New Family.

I know that you're too young right now to have email up there buddy, but you have other ways to communicate with us all down here and we thank you Michael. Keep giving Schering-Plough the ability to continue finding drugs to kill cancer growth.

I must sign off now, or your Mom and Dad are going to yell at me for keeping you up so late, Good night.
Scott Milliman.

978-0-595-36602-6
0-595-36602-3